Colon By Design

Overcoming The Stigma Of Colon Sickness and Unlocking True Colon Health™

First Ed  I0103087

Jenny Berkeley, RN, CHN

BESTSELLING AUTHOR

Copyrights & Digital License

The purpose of this book and this series is to educate. It is sold with the understanding that the publisher and author shall have neither liability nor responsibility for any injury caused or alleged to be caused directly or indirectly by the information contained within this book. Where every effort has been made to ensure accuracy, the book's contents should not be construed as medical advice or a substitute for qualified medical advice. Statements regarding the nutritional content of foods were taken from a variety of sources and may be subject to change.

Each person's health is unique. Seek truth, seek a qualified professional to help guide you, but always follow your heart.

Publisher:
CM BERKELEY MEDIA GROUP
Ontario, Canada
First Edition

Digital ISBN: 978-0-9868018-5-3
Print ISBN: 978-0-9868018-6-0

Copyright

Digital Edition License Notes

Holistic Health Nurse Series™ Books

Volume 1: Eating4Eternity: Unlock Your Holistic Health Lifestyle™

Ever felt that you are suffering prematurely from lifestyle diseases such as pain in the body, weight gain, constipation, tiredness, and what doctors call "getting old"? This book will help you unlock a holistic health lifestyle that your body is aching for. Available in Print and Digital at
http://amzn.to/wagvHC

Volume 2: Sweet Raw Desserts: Life Is Sweet Raw™

An amazing assortment of mouth-watering raw desserts for the whole family. No cooking! You'll love these rawfood recipes more than their traditional, cooked counterparts. Available in Print and Digital at http://amzn.to/MYer1e

Volume 3: Colon By Design: Overcoming the Stigma of Colon Sickness and Unlocking True Colon Health™

Jenny's passion for colon health has driven her to craft this excellent guide for anyone interested in keep their colon healthy. In the years to come, it is almost certain that this book will become the authority for ordinary people to turn to for health and wellness education. Available in Print and Digital at http://amzn.to/MYer1e

Volume 4: Fresh Food4Life™: The Case For Taking Back Control of Your Food and Empowering Your Family and Community.

This next volume in the series takes a look at the most fundamental right of human beings on the planet. It is the right to have access to good quality food to eat and live. Available in Print and Digital at http://amzn.to/Q8Zaf5

Volume 5: Jenny's 99 Heath Quotes To Empower Your Life

This book is for your soul. Fill with quotes to motivate you, to comfort you, and to help you along with path. Look for it online in 2014.

Volume 6: Jenny's DETOX For Health
Detox has become a buzzword. Learn from this holistic health nurse the core of detox and how to help your body. Available by the end of 2014.

Volume 7: Healthy Lunch Box For Kids
The healthy lunchbox is one of Jenny's passions. She wants parents to give their kids a great start by starting with the foods their kids eat. Available by the end of 2014.

Volume 8: Juice Fasting For Vitality
Juicing is one of the greatest things you can do for your body. This book helps you understand why and how to make it a part of your life. Coming soon.

Volume 9: Avoiding The Coming Medical Tsunami
For years, Jenny's been sounding an alarm on what's coming based on her medical experience, her research, and her insider knowledge of hospitals where she has worked. Coming soon.

Volume 10: Holistic Approach To Oral Care
You won't believe what people do to their teeth and gums. Jenny tackles the topic from a holistic health point of view. Coming soon.

* * * * *

Forget the hype about writing your book in 3 hours, or 1 day, or even one week. You know that quality takes times, don't you? Learn our system to becoming a published author in 90 days? CM Berkeley Media Group has an online training program to help anyone aspiring to achieve this dream. Find out more about it and realize your dream at cmberkeleymediagroup.com/writeyourbookin90days/

* * * * *

Dedication

This book is dedicated to everyone who has experienced some form of colon issues. Having been a nurse in the emergency room for over 23 years, I have seen patients come in to the hospital in pain and sorrow. I have been there feeling it with you all.

The saying that an ounce of prevention is worth a pound of cure is never more true than in today's hectic world. And this book is dedicated to every searcher for the truth of life and abundant health and wellness.

It is my hope that all my readers, like you, will take back control of their health destiny.

* * * * *

Acknowledgements

This book, and indeed, this series would not have been possible without the hard work and dedication of all those who support the concepts of good health, a cruelty-free world, justice and equity, and love.

Writing one book is difficult enough, but writing a series of books is more consuming and challenging than a person realizes. Only another seasoned author truly appreciates the effort and the pain. Many writers have remarked that writing is an all-consuming mistress who desires no other competition for her attention. That seems so true at times.

On that note, we express our love and gratitude for all those on our team who keep the ship afloat and all do their parts to make this possible.

Jean Booth, our editor

CM BERKELEY MEDIA GROUP, our publisher

Dr. Brian Clement, my friend and mentor

My friends and family

Trusted Colleagues, our advanced readers

Thank you, all.

* * * * *

The Next Volume in the Series

This is the third book in the series. I decided to publish this book because of my belief that colon health is one of the most vital areas of human health that is overlooked.

This book is written with the purpose of helping the reader understand how vitally important it is to have a clean, well functioning colon. It is really an appeal to the mind of the reader to relate to their inner gut. Other books in my series appeal to your head or your taste-buds, but this one looks to your gut.

It is my hope in writing this book that you will be able to connect the dots and see where conventional thinking has its shortfalls.

I also want you to be able to put a proper system in place, whereby you can enjoy the best of life with assurance that you are doing your part.

* * * * *

Contents

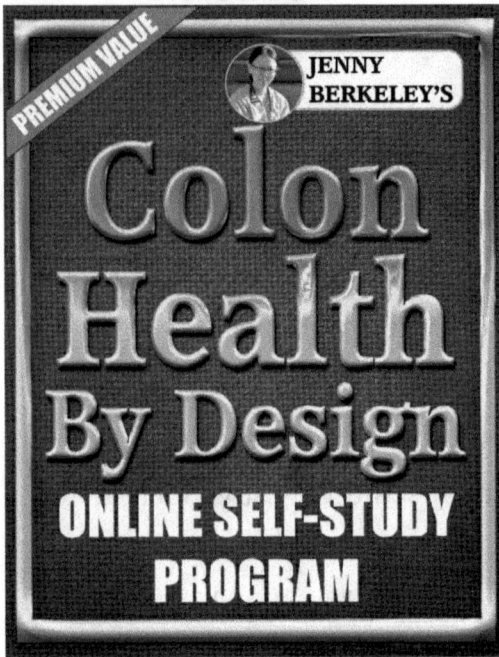

If you need a bit more help understanding your colon, then consider the online self-study program to help you really get this. Because we know that everyone learns in different ways and formats. Check it out at:

http://eating4eternity.org

Diseases of the Colon

Chapter 1

* * *

"The time is always right to do what is right." - Martin Luther King Jr.

"Colon health is one of the most important topics to the human being, yet it is something of a taboo topic. For health to flourish, we must overcome that taboo and look to real care of our colons." - Jenny Berkeley, RN, Health Educator

* * *

When I work in a hospital emergency room I am very mindful of all the patients who check in. From my personal observations, I have seen that many patients come in with some sort of digestive or bowel problem. And for some the situation becomes a revolving door to the local hospital emergency room.

When I started nursing over 23 years ago, I was more likely to see a person in their middle age to senior years come in with bowel conditions. Now I see people coming into the emergency room younger and younger with diseases of the colon and digestive tract.

Let's look at a few dis-eases of the digestive system.

Constipation

Constipation is an affliction of the lower part of the digestive tract. It is prevalent in the large intestines and colon. It comes in three levels. There is mild constipation, severe constipation, and chronic constipation.

Most times people do not come into the hospital for mild constipation. They try to treat this themselves by taking general over-the-counter stool softeners or even extra fiber. This can provide some relief for some people, but if it is not accompanied by proper dietary changes, then there's always a risk of increasing severity.

For severe constipation I have seen people stumble into the emergency room in pain over the years. At this juncture all their attempts at self treatment have failed. And I would suspect this is because they only had a tiny bit of knowledge as their basis for working with their body. And the approach was very narrow in focus instead of a holistic approach, which I tend to recommend to my clients.

With severe and painful constipation, we have to prepare a patient for the doctor. The interview with a patient is to determine the extent of the situation. Sometimes the doctor may recommend we use an enema to try to get moisture into the region.

If that fails to bring relief, then the doctor may have to use his or her hand to reach into the rectum and manually take out the impacted stool. It is a very unpleasant and painful procedure.

Many times the patient will be discharged feeling a bit better after the blockage is cleared, only to return a few days or weeks later. That is why I call it a revolving-door disease of the digestive system.

Chronic constipation may have life-altering consequences for the patient. This may include removal of sections of the colon, and the use of a colostomy bag. At this point the disease is considered irreversible and the damage to the colon is permanent.

IBS or Crohn's Disease

This is an affliction of the small intestines. Irritable bowel syndrome is a disease that has been characterized as one of the most perplexing and annoying of the gastrointestinal conditions. This dis-ease of the small intestine is one that is characterized by severe pain, loss of appetite, debilitating discomfort, and loose stool.

This disease is often difficult because the doctors have difficulty trying to pin down the specific cause of the situation in order to address it. And this means that many patients without the knowledge of a holistic health and wellness approach to diet and lifestyle, will continue doing the same things that are contributing to the disease.

My very good friend, Paul Nison, was afflicted with this disease in his youth. It was extremely severe and his doctors had told him that it was incurable. He would be doomed to spend the rest of his life with this pain and suffering whenever he ate. But he never gave up hope.

At the time, Paul was living in New York City with a high-paced and stressful lifestyle. He also admits he had a terrible view of dietary wellness. He ate all sorts of junk food and the typical Standard American Diet (SAD).

Paul gave up his high-stress lifestyle in New York City and moved to Florida, where he hoped the change would help heal his condition. This was very helpful to Paul, but he still had his affliction to deal with. It was only when he discovered the Hippocrates Health Institute in Florida that his life truly began to turn around.

Paul had switched to a living foods diet. Paul had also removed the stress from his life. And Paul was now approaching life from a holistic point of view. He was living life. Paul eventually totally reversed the disease and wrote a book about his journey. I highly recommend his book.

I'll put forward four possibilities that work together in this disease and related diseases of the intestine. These are:

1. Lifestyle/Emotional Stress
2. Poor Diet & Nutrition

3. Poor Intestinal Flora
4. Poor Elimination

It is my belief that all four of these factors, working to varying degrees, create conditions of disease within the intestinal tract. I'll discuss these more later on in the chapters.

Ulcerative Colitis

Ulcerative colitis is a form of inflammatory bowel disease in which the sores develop in the lining of the colon and rectum. These sores bleed and produce pus. The colon averages about 5 feet long. The irritation can be anywhere along that length.

Gastroesophageal Reflux Disease (GERD/Acid Reflux)

Acid reflux is commonly considered a chronic condition which afflicts the patient. It is characterized by heartburn which is mild in the beginning but soon progresses to severe. This is due to the digestive juices from the stomach escaping upward into the oesophagus. One reason given for this situation is that the sphincter muscle and the base of the oesophagus are malfunctioning and unable to close fully during digestion.

This inability to close fully allows the stomach acid to rise into the oesophagus which creates the burning sensation along the upper digestive tract. Sometimes the acid makes its way all the way up to the back of the throat where the patient can taste the acidity.

When the disease is still quite mild, patients may consider the use of over-the-counter antacids to try to combat this condition. This only provides temporary relief and over time the condition gets worse. As it progresses, the patient will seek a doctor for a stronger, prescription-strength antacid. Once a person begins down this route, it is highly unlikely that they will stop taking these prescription antacids. It will become a lifelong habit. Once they stop taking it the symptoms of the condition will return severely.

However looking at this symptom only and treating this symptom does not get to the underlying root of the problem. In order to get to the root, one must take a holistic approach towards health and wellness.

The stomach is only acidic when it is involved in digesting food. When the stomach is empty, it should not be acidic.

One person I was working with had such a severe case of acid reflux that he would have to sleep at night with his upper body tilted upward. We worked together to try to understand what he was doing that was contributing to the ongoing progression of his disease. When he modified his diet and lifestyle, he began to see relief.

Again, it was taking a holistic approach to his life that helped him to move out of this state and make improvements.

Leaky Gut Syndrome (LGS)

This is another common gastrointestinal condition where the intestine wall becomes filled with tiny holes. These holes allow undigested food to leak into the blood. When this happens, it triggers an autoimmune response in your body. Your body sees the undigested food particles as a toxin in the blood stream and you experience a type of allergic reaction to the food. Leaky gut syndrome can also be responsible for nutritional deficiency and poor absorption of food.

Remember, the intestine is a muscular tube. For a hole to develop in this tube, it means that a large portion of cells had to die in that area. The question to ask is, what killed a group of cells in a specific region in the intestine? In the movie, Genetic Roulette, several learned individuals talk about the linkage between genetically modified foods and the leaky gut syndrome. Of particular interest is that children with LGS who developed allergies to foods, eventually were able to eat those same foods as long as they were organic. Whenever the conventional/GMO food was reintroduced, the symptoms came back. I touch on the concept of GMO in a later chapter and why I believe it is not beneficial to human health and your intestinal and colon health.

People with LGS tend to experience some mineral deficiencies as the inflammation in the region interferes with the absorption of certain minerals. These include magnesium, zinc, copper, and calcium.

In order to address LGS in a holistic way, one has to remove whatever is killing the cells of the intestine as well as provide the body with elements it needs to repair and thrive. This means cutting out the food which is the conduit for the toxins killing your intestinal wall cells, allowing your body time to heal, then reintroducing the organic versions of those foods at a much later time.

The Four Factors which impact intestinal dis-eases

As you can probably tell by now, I am a strong advocate of taking a holistic approach to health and wellness. Every disease does not happen in isolation. They are a combination of a variety of forces working together to achieve the outcome. Thus, for anyone wanting the path to a healthier life, only a truly holistic approach is the way to approach dis-ease.

While looking at disease of the colon and intestinal tract, we want to consider the following four factors:

1. Poor Lifestyle/Emotional Stress
2. Poor Diet & Nutrition
3. Poor Intestinal Flora
4. Poor Elimination

Poor Lifestyle & Emotional Stress

Too many people are living in this modern-day society with complete disregard to the natural and biological laws which govern our existence. This daily disregard forms the basis of what is called a habit. Over time this habit becomes strongly entrenched within every fibre of a person's being.

Take, for example, the issue of sleep. Our bodies are designed to rest during the night. In many parts of the world and depending on the time of year, it may get dark at 6 p.m., 7 p.m., or 8 p.m.. Thus we should be in bed by that time. However, electricity and television have altered many of our natural sleep patterns. After all, people are just getting warmed up at 8 p.m.. All of the television shows that come on after the news are called prime time programming. In reality, this is the prime time to get to bed and start resting your body, not to be staying up to watch television.

Another example is the high-stress jobs that many people are working in today. Even jobs which should be low stress become high stress when people are sleep deprived, overworked and underpaid. Many people are on the verge of workplace burnout and they don't even recognize it.

Like with Paul Nison, it will take some major life illness or catastrophe to jolt them into reassessing their lifestyle choices. And yet, because they are operating from a limited knowledge base, they make the best decision they can, but it does not produce the optimum result or the results are much slower than they should be.

In order to break this cycle, some people need to work with a qualified individual who can guide them along the path to holistic health and wellness. They need a coach and an advocate. This should be a person who has a background in the field of medicine plus knowledge of natural health, diet, and other health and wellness principles. The best person to be a guide is one who looks at the person as a whole being and practices a holistic health approach.

Working with such a person to get to the root cause of the lifestyle and emotional stresses can help move you quickly along the path of holistic health and wellness.

Poor Diet & Nutrition

Diet and nutrition are two other areas that are contributing factors in the progression of diseases of the intestines and colon. There is an Egyptian proverb that says one quarter of what you eat keeps you alive and the other three-quarters keeps your doctor alive. It may sound humorous, but too many people are consuming a diet that is poorly structured with little to no real nutritional value.

Take for example the number of times a day a person should eat. I've actually read that some people suggest eating six meals a day or about every two hours. I could not believe that nonsense when I read it. The first question that comes to my mind is, when does your stomach rest on such a routine? It is completely unsustainable to abusively overwork your digestive system in that manner. Depending on the type of meals that people consume, there is a tendency to feel tired after a meal. There are so many processes involved in moving food from your mouth to your colon that I would warn people away from that frequency of eating.

An average sedentary person need only eat 2 to 3 times a day. And those meals should be at least four hours apart with no snacking or any meal in between. This will give your digestive system sufficient time to work with your meal and allow your stomach to get some rest before the next meal. It also gives the digestive system sufficient time to digest the food without restarting the process.

Even a simple thing like chewing gum after your meal is a destructive habit. Let's say you eat lunch from noon to 1 p.m. Then as you finish your lunch, you begin to chew a stick of gum to help "wash your mouth with saliva." And let's say your gum was long lasting – until 2 p.m. What you have done by chewing for an hour is re-set the clock on your digestion and you basically told your body that lunch ended at 2 p.m. instead of 1 p.m. And this is when your stomach processes begin to work.

Remember my client with acid reflux? After he had eaten, I noticed him taking out a stick of gum. I questioned him about that habit. And I immediately advised him to put a stop to it.

Like every muscle in your body, you need time to work, and rest. And your stomach muscles need their rest periods too.

If you find that you are frequently hungry when eating 2 or 3 meals a day, it could be habit hunger or you may be lacking in some vital nutrients which is causing your body to trigger the hunger sensation.

A holistic approach would involve fixing the negative habits associated with eating in addition to incorporating a richer, nutrient dense, whole-food plant-based diet.

Poor Intestinal Flora

Within your colon, you need a healthy balance of good bacteria and bad bacteria. This is because each kind of bacteria serves a specific function in the digestion process. When you have more of the bad bacteria than the good bacteria, it throws your system out of whack.

And there are any number of factors which can contribute to this imbalance. One may be eating a diet that promotes the growth of bad bacteria while stunting the growth of good bacteria. There may be some genetic contamination of your bacteria due to the consumption of GMOs. Or even going through a series of antibiotic treatments can kill your internal bacteria and cause an imbalance in the system.

Restoring this area of the colon back to health would require you to take a probiotic supplement which can help replenish the bacteria along with eating a diet that is conducive to the optimal environment for this good bacteria.

I discuss probiotics in greater detail in the chapter on supplements and digestive health.

Poor Elimination

The last major factor that contributes to the overall ill-health of the digestive system and the colon is the speed at which toxins are eliminated. When toxins move too slowly from your body, it is called constipation. And when they move too fast, it is called diarrhoea. Neither of these conditions is desirable. A process of elimination of waste from the colon should be regular and timely.

People develop poor elimination techniques due to improper posture, improper diet, and improper training and conditioning, I talk about posture training and conditioning in the chapter on the proper elimination protocol.

It is important to begin to work on the right way to eliminate your food waste in order to maintain a healthy colon.

Chapter Summary

In this chapter of the book we discussed a few diseases of the colon. I also gave you a few insights based on taking a holistic approach to our overall health and wellness.

* * * * *

Proper Elimination Protocol
Chapter 2

* * *

"Courage is the most important of all virtues, because without it we can't practice any other virtue with consistency." - Maya Angelou

"Consistency and regularity in your bowel movements is nurtured each day or weakened each day. Either you employ a proper protocol which strengthens your colon or you practice an improper protocol which weakens your colon. Then people wonder why they need adult diapers at age 70." - Jenny Berkeley, RN, Health Educator

* * *

Why is regular elimination necessary?

We all eat every day. Eating is probably one of the most fundamental things we do in our lives. Think about it, when a baby exits the womb, the baby breathes, cries, is held by the mother, and then placed on the breast to suck.

Babies, toddlers, children, teens, and adults all have different biological functions and timings as those functions relate to their everyday life. Babies spend more time eating and pooping as their bodies are developing rapidly during the first 12 to 24 months. Children who eat, play, go to school, and have an active lifestyle also have a different pattern of bowel function and elimination. And adults have a different pattern because they exercise more control over their natural functions, sometimes to their own detriment.

Regular elimination of food waste via bowel movements is essential. I remember a discussion with a paediatric doctor one time about an infant. The infant had not had a bowel movement in about 3 to 4 days and the parent was naturally concerned. The paediatrician smiled and indicated that this was perfectly normal and that she had once seen an infant who didn't have a movement for 14 days. The parent in this case did not feel comforted by this statement.

After the parent's persistence, the doctor recommended a glycerin suppository for the infant if the mother still had concerns after another day or so. I'll speak more about colon health and the impact on children in a later chapter.

In the hospital emergency room I have seen patients in terrible pain after only 4 to 6 days of not having a bowel movement. The body has managed to turn the stool into a hard, rock-like object along the intestinal wall, which can be painful.

Regular elimination is therefore very essential to ensuring that the process is not painful and toxins from the body are eliminated in a timely manner and not reabsorbed into the body.

In order to have proper elimination as a regular, routine, biological function, it is important as you grow older to build a proper habit into your lifestyle which will ensure healthy bowel moments.

What are the ingredients needed for bowel movement?

In order to have a bowel movement you need to have all of the following:

○ You need to have a lot of **moisture** inside of your intestinal tract to lubricate and move the food forward along each stage of the digestive process. As we will see in the stages in the chapter on digestion, every input into each area affects the output for that area. And that output is the input for the next stage in the process. Drinking water 30 minutes prior to eating is one way to add some moisture and lubrication to the system.

○ You need to have **plant fibre** in order to add more bulk to the food and help sweep the colon. This must be raw, living food plant fibre, not some powder that is added to a solution and then swallowed. If you are only eating processed, refined foods that break down into a putty consistency, then it requires a lot more water to make this type of texture easily movable along the intestine. Plant-based fibres like those found in fruits, vegetables, and greens, are perfect for moving along the intestine while refined flour food products like breads, pastas, pastries, are not.

○ You must have **the urge to eliminate** via the body's normal peristalsis movement. This urge to go to the toilet is a normal signal of the body to clean out the toxic waste. There are certain times when you can help trigger this urge. In fact, every day upon waking, you can trigger your body to have a bowel movement if you train yourself as a habit and drink water first thing in the morning. If you have been abusing your body for a while by ignoring it, you may have to keep at it to restore the function.

○ You must **immediately respond** to the body's urge so that the body does not delay the waste removal. People can ignore this if they are travelling on a train commute home, or in an important meeting, or are embarrassed to use a person's toilet if they are a guest in their home. The longer a person delays this, the greater the risk of developing constipation or something worse. If you ignore it, your body may decide to wait, but the longer the stool sits in the colon and rectum, the more moisture is eliminated and the harder it becomes.

Form and Function of the Colon

Standing

Is there is a right way or a wrong way to have a bowel movement? Absolutely, yes. Let's consider standing up for example. Can you have a bowel movement standing? Certainly not, under normal conditions. However there have been rare instances where a person was so stressed or scared that they pooped themselves while in a standing or vertical position.

The body is designed functionally to prevent this sort of thing from happening, yet there are instances when the mind can override these safeguards and cause an unexpected outcome in the bowels. We say a person has had an accident when that happens.

Normally, the standing position of the human form causes the sphincter muscle in the rectum to contract and maintain closure to prevent leakage or untimely elimination of fecal matter.

First we can see that standing is an inappropriate form for the process of elimination of food waste from the colon.

Sitting

Is sitting down an appropriate position for elimination of stool from the bowel?

Before we answer this question, let's look at some of the ways in which we use the form of sitting. We sit down to drive an automobile. Should we be having a bowel movement at that time? No, of course not. We sit down in our offices in order to do work. Should we be having a bowel movement at that time? No, of course not. We sit down to watch television or surf the Internet. Should we be having a bowel movement at that time? No, of course not. Lastly we sit down to eat. Should we be having a bowel movement at that time? No, of course not.

Sitting down is a wonderful, functional form of the human body, however it is not the form designed by nature for optimum elimination of waste from the colon. Just like standing, you can force yourself to have a bowel movement while sitting, but that does not make it the right way for your long-term health and vitality, especially in the area of colon health.

Based on my years of experience and my personal studies on this topic, I can let you know that forcing yourself to eliminate in the sitting position day after day, month after month, year after year, will eventually lead you to your senior years and the need to wear adult disposable diapers once you have ruined the sphincter muscle at your anus.

Squatting

Is squatting the ideal position for proper bowel movements and elimination of waste food from the colon? The answer is resoundingly yes. This may upset many toilet makers because the design of the conventional toilet is flawed in that it will create abnormalities or malfunctions when a person is in their 70s and 80s.

Squatting is still the functional form that nature has designed for the human body to properly and efficiently eliminate waste from the colon. If you look at any two- or three-year old child who has not been potty trained, you will notice that that child will naturally squat when needing to have a bowel movement. When parents "potty train" their children into using the incorrect functional form, i.e., sitting, they are unintentionally setting their children on a path that will lead to colon issues later on in life.

In this current world of abundant knowledge it is about

time that someone sound the alarm about the unintentional harm conventional toilets do because it is forcing the application of the wrong form for a specific function.

The modern toilets used by most western civilizations are designed for ease of use and convenience. Their purpose is to allow a person who is unable or unwilling to squat to sit and defecate. And while it seems to be a convenient solution, it is actually an inconvenient item.

Japanese scientists researched the pressure used by persons sitting on a toilet versus a person squatting to poop. They found that persons squatting were able to defecate quickly with less straining and pressure.

This goes back to our biological design. In the sitting and standing position, the rectum is folded over like a bathroom towel over a towel rack. The puborectal muscle is the "rack." When humans squat, they are at a 35-degree angle, which is the optimum angle to unkink the rectum. When it is unkinked, the fecal matter slides out faster, with less pressure and straining, and more thoroughly. There is little to no matter left behind.

In talks and lectures I give on this topic, it is always harder for the older folks. This is because their bodies have undergone 10, 15, 20 years or more of the improper posture. They find it the most difficult to stretch their calf muscles to squat. They also may have some long-held beliefs that their old way is correct, so their mind is resistant.

However, even the Dr. Oz television show has featured the proper way to squat and a device to help people who have difficulty squatting. I did not like the way it was fleetingly dealt with as a wacky idea that works. But at least it got some mainstream media exposure that way.

In my opinion, the conventional sitting toilet is like where tobacco was in the mid-1950s. Many people, even medical professionals thought smoking was good, but by the year 2000, everyone knew that smoking was bad and the cause of serious health conditions.

People are beginning to wake up. Even Doctor Oz, a mainstream show, has featured this knowledge. However like BIG tobacco bears some responsibility for cancer, conventional toilet makers bear some of the responsibility for diseases of the colon caused by habitual faulty defecation via the use of their equipment. It's like a worker using a workspace that was known to cause injury like carpel tunnel syndrome. If people are using a toilet at home and work that is known to contribute to colon ill-health, then changes need to be made.

On a macro level

On the governmental, macro level, there needs to be a re-visitation of regulations regarding the installation of toilets. Since those regulations are designed to favour sitting toilets, they are favouring ill colon health. Everything from workplace stalls to home bathrooms needs to be revisited.

On a personal level

While we are waiting for the government to get with the program, we can purchase devices to assist with attaining the squatting position on the toilet. Or if you live in an Eastern country that has access to a squatting toilet, then get one for yourself.

Making sure that you continue to squat today and your loved ones learn why squatting is important is the best thing you can do for your personal colon health and that of your family.

The information I've given you here is ancient yet futuristic because society lost this knowledge. Take it now and make it part of your essence.

Chapter Summary

In this chapter we covered the components that go into making a bowel movement. We also looked at the functional aspects of pooping to understand why so many people simply have it backwards. This is one instance where you want to be different from the crowd so that you are not suffering with colon illness in 15 to 20 years.

Chapter References

Sakakibara et al. Influence of Body Position on Defecation in Humans.

* * * * *

Water and Colon Health

Chapter 3

* * *

"Water not only sustains life but protects life." - Sang Whang, author of Reverse Aging.

Water is the miracle solution in your body. Like water is life to our planet, so too it is life to our cells. We must respect this water and cherish it in order to thrive both within and without. - Jenny Berkeley, RN, Certified Holistic Nutritionist

* * *

I am very passionate about the influence of water on the human body and the linkage to our health and vitality. Over the years, I have blogged and lectured about the importance of water in reversing certain states of dis-ease within the body as well as preventing the onset of certain states of dis-ease.

It is important for you to understand that water is one of the key factors to human life. When we are born, our bodies are made up of about 90% water, and at the end of life, our bodies are around 50% water. For optimal health and vitality, we must ensure that our bodies are well hydrated each and every day.

Water is a form of magical solution. Water has the ability to dissolve nutrients, mineral salts, and certain fats. When people come into the emergency room, I ask them how much water they've had to drink in the past 24 hours. The average answer is 1 or 2 cups. Then they begin to tell me about coffee, teas, juices, or other liquid foods they have ingested which they consider to be water.

The distinction between water and non-water

It seems to me that over the years people have come to the false understanding that anything that contains water counts toward your water intake. This erroneous assumption is what is leading many Canadians and many people across the world into a state of chronic dehydration.

Now I am going to give you a re-education about water.

Water is pure water or mineral water. That is all! Water is not fruit juice. It is not coffee. It is not regular or diet sodas. I, as well as many health professionals in the area of health and wellness, consider those things to be liquid foods.

Think about this for a moment. A soup contains mostly water with some solid ingredients boiled down into the soup. If you drink the soup water only, you know that you are getting the dissolved nutrients from the soup ingredients into your body. You are "eating" soup as your meal.

This is the same way to consider all fruit and vegetable juices. They are liquid foods just as the soup is a food. It is also the same reason that diet sodas, coffee drinks, and any other kind of drink that is not pure water is a liquid food.

You simply cannot consider a liquid food as part of your daily water intake. Your body is much smarter than you are and knows that it is food even if you call it water with your mind.

Why is this distinction even necessary?

It is important to make the distinction because of the way your body reacts when these food items are ingested as opposed to when water is ingested.

You see, the sodas, the juices, the caffeinated beverages, and all the other types of drinks contain starches or sugars that the body has to digest. They may also contain proteins and fats if milk is added, for example. They may also contain stimulants like caffeine. All of these things trigger the digestive response within the body.

So never again think of a drink that contains water as counting toward your water intake. It does not count toward your water intake. A more accurate way to think of it is as counting toward your meal/food intake.

These are liquid meals and you are "eating" for the purpose of digestion.

Why is it important that I understand this?

It is important because the process of digestion is one that requires the use of vast quantities of water within the stomach and the small intestine.

Now here is the simplicity and the genius of the entire matter.

When you are thirsty and you drink these liquid foods, you force the body to take water out of the general circulation to put it into the digestive process. When you do this, you are adding additional stress and strain to your blood, your lymphatic system, your kidneys, and every other organ of the body.

You see, the body is a complete system and all the processes are interconnected. Because all of the blood, tissues, and organs are all fed by the same river of life, that is, water, flowing through this enclosed system, when anything is done to disrupt the natural water balance in the body, then you will have dire consequences.

Here's a curious point to ponder: Ever thought about why it is that when patients are rushed into the hospital emergency room, one of the first things that is done is to insert a needle into the vein and run an intravenous (IV) solution? This solution is water and a bit of salt, otherwise called a saline solution. Why do you think that this solution is run directly into the bloodstream when a patient arrives at the ER? Based on what has been discussed earlier, I'll let you draw the conclusion.

That is why, I can 9 out of 10 times be certain that patients arriving in the hospital have had less than two litres of pure water in a day. One cup or two of pure water is grossly inadequate for even survival, let alone thriving.

Implications of Improper Water Intake

Dr. Timothy Brantley makes an interesting statement in his book,

"The condition and state of the circulating fluids in our bodies is a main factor in determining our overall health, which is completely dependent on the quality and the amount of water we feed it daily. In fact, each bio-chemical reaction inside our bodies is totally dependent on the quality, structure and amount of water that our cells, tissues, and organs constantly receive." [Dr. Brantley book, pg 115)

Dr. Brantley also goes on to discuss a patient of his. Kristin suffered from chronic dehydration accompanied by irregular heartbeat and pain in her left arm for 10 years. Dr. Brantley says that Kristin, like many of his other patients, had tried many different treatments with no success before finally arriving at his clinic. She was a woman who now lived in fear of her sickness. She was only in her mid-40s, but living the lifestyle of an 80-year old, afraid of having a heart attack.

Kristin went to see Dr. Brantley because of the reputation of his herbal formulas. She was hopeful that he would be able to whip up a suitable concoction to cure her particular ailment. At that point she was willing to try any potion or lotion since nothing else worked.

After Dr. Brantley spent some time assessing her, his recommendation was that she drink more water. Kristin said she would drink more water, then proceeded to ask for her heart formula. When Dr. Brantley told her that she did not need any formulation, but simply needed to drink more water, she was confused and dumbfounded.

She retorted, "You've got to be kidding me! You mean to tell me that I've seen everyone in Los Angeles to help correct my skipped heartbeats and all you can tell me is to drink water?"

She left his clinic in a daze but was determined to try this protocol. Some weeks later she phoned Dr. Brantley to tell him that her skipped heartbeats were gone.

This is an example of a person who suffered needlessly for about ten years, and spent tons of money and time searching for anything that could help her. In the end, the solution was something so simple, yet so important to life on this planet, that she was amazed when she saw it did work.

Water is 70% of the adult human being. I want you to recognize that water is an essential part of your colon health strategy. If you are not taking in enough water, it will impact your colon and every other area of your body.

But our topic is the colon, so I'll go on to how improper intake impacts your colon. In my lectures on colon health, I give people an overview of the colon and digestion.

Here are the basic steps:
1. You put food (solid or liquid) into your mouth.
2. Sensors in your mouth tell the brain that food is coming into the digestive system.
3. Your stomach begins to moisten itself and create the necessary digestive juices.
4. As the food enters your stomach, more liquid is added based on the amount of food.

5. All food in the stomach is liquefied.
6. The liquid "soup" is sent into the small intestine.
7. More juices are manufactured by the body to neutralize the acidity and make the soup less viscous, that is, a "runny soup."
8. Nutrients are absorbed from the "runny soup" in the small intestines.
9. The leftover soup water is sent to the large intestines (colon).
10. Water is recycled (extracted) before the solid waste is eliminated.

Here's a little more detail.

Step 1

Now you can see that whether you put in a liquid meal or a solid meal, you are still putting a meal into your mouth. Sometimes people mistake signs of thirst for hunger and they put more food in their body when they need to drink water.

Steps 2, 3 & 4

At this point your body is turning up the digestive system. The digestive juices are manufactured on an as-needed basis. Water is one of the ingredients used to manufacture your digestive juices. These manufactured juices are then secreted by the stomach walls into the stomach. The body takes water out of the general circulation to deal with this digestion. The amount of water required to digest your food is directly proportional to the amount of food you consume AND the degree of processing your food has undergone. See more on this in the chapter on digestion and colon health.

Steps 5, 6 & 7

At this point, water has only been removed from the general circulation of your body to make digestion possible. For a person who is already dehydrated, the brain now has to manage all the vital organs of the body and the blood on a dangerously low amount of water.

Can you guess what happens in some instances? The onset of ITIS! This is a slang term, not a medical term, but it identifies clearly what happens to dehydrated people after a meal. They feel sleepy and dopey after eating. Those who are not at work have the luxury of going to sleep for two or three hours. This is a necessary survival mechanism for the dehydrated person. The brain says, "okay, we don't have enough water in this body so, we'll put the body into rest mode so that water can be used in digestion, then when we begin extracting the water, we'll wake up the body."

Isn't the human body amazing? I love it! If you know someone who always MUST sleep after eating, then they are chronically dehydrated.

Steps 8, 9 & 10
At this point, the nutrients from the meal are being extracted and afterward the body will attempt to reclaim the water from the large intestine. And because the person is already dehydrated and does not drink enough water daily, the body will aggressively extract the water from the colon.

When the body attempts to aggressively extract the water, can you guess what happens to the individual?

That person begins to have trouble with their colon. At first the stool may seem compacted like a log. And over time, as the situation goes from bad to worse, the person will see hard "bird pellets" coming out of the stool. That is a sign there is not even enough moisture to hold the poop together. The colon is super aggressively pulling out water and the person is having infrequent bowel movements.

Finally one day, the person is driving into the hospital parking lot in pain. Crawling to get to the emergency room. Who knows the thoughts going through their mind? Perhaps they are questioning God at that point, or if they didn't believe in God, hoping that there is a god to make the pain go away. They get to the emergency room howling in pain for the doctors and nurses to help them. But they have to take a number and wait in the waiting room like everyone else.

When the doctor finally sees the patient, he assesses the condition of the patient's stomach. And if this is a first time, maybe prescribes some laxatives for the patient to go home to take. They go home and try the laxatives. They still never modify their water-intake habit. And then within a week or two, they are back into the emergency room howling and complaining of the same pain.

The situation turns the hospital emergency room into a kind of revolving door for the patient who is ignorant of the workings of their body and the vitally important impact of water on colon health. And at upwards of $400 a visit, it can be a very costly thing. Canadians should be truly thankful that universal healthcare is provided. Yet, I feel there is some wastage of taxpayers' money when a patient has to come in several times for the same dis-ease state of the body.

In the United States and other countries where people have to pay for their health care costs, you will see more open-minded individuals, ready to search for a cheaper way to resolve basic things. They recognize that hospitals are for the really serious items because every visit translates to money out of their pocket.

Dr. Shinya's Experience Briefly Explained

Most people do not know of Dr. Shinya, yet many people should be grateful to him. He was the inventor of the colonscope in 1967. Back in his early days of the medical profession, the only way to tell what was happening in someone's colon was to cut open their abdomen (laparotomy) and look inside their colon.

Due to Dr. Shinya's invention, patients now only need

to lie down while the scope is inserted into their rectum. It is still an unpleasant procedure, but it beats getting cut open any day. His technique for removing polyps from the colon is called the Shinya Technique.

He is a highly respected medical doctor who works out of New York and Japan. Over his decades of examining the colons of Americans and Japanese, he has made some amazing observations.

He noted that the Standard American Diet (SAD), has had a terrible impact on the colon of patients he examined. He states (pg 20),

"American colons were clearly firmer and shorter than Japanese colons. In addition to the lumen being narrower, ring-like bumps had formed in certain areas as though they were toed off with rubber bands. There were also many diverticulosis and frequent accumulations of stagnant stool."

He further goes on to state (Ibid),

"Such deterioration of intestinal conditions results not only in disease like colon cancer, colonic polyps, and diverticulosis. Many people with unhealthy intestines in fact become ill with lifestyle-related diseases, such as fibroids, hypertension (high blood pressure), arteriosclerosis, heart disease, obesity, breast cancer, prostate cancer, and diabetes. When your intestines are unhealthy, your body is gradually weakened from the inside."

As part of Dr. Shinya's treatment protocol, it is mandatory for the patient to increase their water level intake to the levels that he recommends to help cleanse the colon.

Do you understand now how vitally important it is to make the connection between a healthy colon and overall health, wellness and vitality?

So what is the incentive for Canadians or anyone living in a country with universal healthcare coverage to maintain a healthy and hydrated colon?

In one word, TIME.

Your time is infinitely valuable. Would you like to spend hours in an emergency room waiting for a doctor to see you? Would you like to spend hours, days, months or years in pain, suffering, and in fear of some state of dis-ease instead of living those same moments of life in joy, happiness, and gratitude?

My website, http://www.eating4eternity.org has on online study course based on this book that can enable you to become a master of your colon again.

Chapter Summary

In this chapter, I have given you the simplest insight into how your colon functions with respect to the need for water. You have seen from the experiences of Dr. Brantley and Dr. Shinya, two very respected MDs, their experiences with water and with the colon. My own experiences with water have shown that by increasing the intake of water, we can have better elimination of the stool, reduce the tendency for the ITIS that happens after meals, and have a better, more vibrant quality of life.

Chapter References

Brantley, Timothy. The Cure: Heal Your Body, Save Your Life.
Shinya, Hiromi. The Enzyme Factor.
Berkeley, Jenny. Blog Post

* * * * *

Colon Hydrotherapy and Colon Health

Chapter 4

* * *

"Esteem yourself with men of good quality if you esteem your own reputation, for 'tis better to be alone than in bad company." - George Washington

"The battle in your colon rages on daily. And each day you support either the good side or the bad side by your dietary choices. There is no neutral ground. Thus it is your duty to choose to support the good side by making the right choices." - Jenny Berkeley, RN, Health Educator

* * *

Did you know...

According to one study of bowel cancer patients between 2010 and 2011, a little over one-fifth of the 29,000 cancer patients recorded were admitted to the hospital ER. Of those admitted, one-third had colon cancer that was too far gone for surgical intervention. And of those who had surgery, 11% died within 90 days.[1]

A "dirty" colon leads to increased risks of all manner of diseases and most especially cancer.

What is colon hydrotherapy?

Colon hydrotherapy is an approach to cleansing the colon via the use of water to flush the colon. It dates back to ancient Egypt where they believed that sickness in the body and the shortening of a person's lifespan was attributed to the build-up of toxins in the colon and the rotting of uneliminated food inside the gut. This was later expanded on by the

Greeks who also thought colon hydrotherapy to be beneficial.

Your colon is the body's sewer system. Proper elimination of food matter which has been left over from the digestive process is essential as a tool in the pursuit of holistic health in your body. If you have not considered a colon cleanse or have never had one in your life, then it is important to speak to a qualified practitioner about the potential for having one done.

The Benefits

Colon hydrotherapy is not a happy or pleasant thing to experience the first few times. Just ask any patient who has had to go into the hospital to have a colonoscopy done. The patient has to drink a horrible tasting solution (a laxative) the day before, along with lots of water in order to cause the patient to have diarrhoea and thus flush out the colon. It can cause abdominal cramping, irritation of the anus, and leave patients with an unpleasant feeling overall. This is not a colon irrigation treatment.

The benefit of colon hydrotherapy is that it uses water applied directly to the colon and large intestine without the use of the laxative solution taken orally. For a patient, this means no "sour stomach" feeling, greatly reduced cramping, and more hydration to the colon wall due to water being used to irrigate the colon. The use of a large volume of water (sometimes 18L or more) flowing in and out of the colon allows for a much more thorough cleaning than would be possible by the patient simply drinking two litres of water with a laxative solution.

And by filling the colon tubes with water, the treatment gently expands the muscles of the wall and causes the muscle to contract and squeeze the water out. This gentle expansion and contraction, combined with the volume of water circulating in the colon can allow for a greater ability to dislodge stool that was not moving freely.

This is strictly the mechanical benefits of having a colon hydrotherapy/irrigation done.

The Colon in a Hospital Setting

Working in the hospital emergency room, I have seen countless number of patients come into the hospital complaining of constipation, whether mild or severe. The doctor will have to assess the patient, but before he or she gets there, we nurses have to do a preliminary question-and-answer to try to determine all the details for the doctor.

Sometimes a patient may have not had a bowel movement for close to a week and may be experiencing discomfort. After the doctor assesses the patient he/she may advise the patient to take a laxative or stool softener to loosen or dislodge the impacted matter. This is if the situation is not too serious by the doctor's assessment.

Sometimes the situation may be worse and the patient may be howling in pain because the rock-hard stool refuses to move. Then the doctor may advise us to get out an enema bag and administer a water treatment for the patient. This bag only has a 1.5L capacity and is administered once to the patient. Then the patient has to sit on the toilet (wrong form for function) and try to flush out the hard stool.

In the most severe cases, the patient may have to lie on her side while the doctor inserts her hand into the anus to dig out the rock-hard fecal matter. This is a most unpleasant and painful experience for the patient.

The Concerns

Those who are against the idea of colon irrigation or who call it quackery have concerns about it being done unless it is done for reasons related to a medical procedure like a colonscopy or some removal of polyps in the colon.

Here are some of the concerns the nay-sayers have against a colonscopy:

- It is an ancient technique (from ancient Egypt and ancient Greece), not really valid in today's modern community.
- There is little scientific evidence to prove the validity of claims.
- There is a lot of anecdotal evidence that it works.
- There are risks of injury to the colon.
- There are risks of electrolyte imbalance in the colon.
- There is a risk of dependency on the procedure.

I'll address each of the above concerns as I believe that you need to hear both sides of the story in order to make an informed decision about whether you want to find out more about hydrotherapy as a tool for your health and wellness.

The ancient technique reason against colon irrigation is one that is a bit discriminatory and irrational like most forms of discrimination. Just because something is old, does not necessarily mean that it is bad or invalid in today's modern society. For example, the principles of medical quarantine and hygiene can be traced back to those ancient teachings as well.

The absence of scientific evidence to prove the validity of colon irrigation to help reduce or eliminate any medical condition. The scientific evidence means a scientific study done with human test subjects. In the absence of clinical studies, one need only examine the hundreds of thousands of colon irrigation treatments done around the world. Of course, if a person were looking specifically for colon irrigation to cure a specific disease, then it would be difficult to find as most people use multiple therapies when treating their condition. One could argue that there is no scientific evidence that bathing can cure any disease, yet we all bathe regularly. At some point common sense needs to prevail. Also note that the Hippocrates Health Institute in West

Palm Beach, Florida has over 50 years of data on humans who have received their treatments, including colon irrigation.

There is a lot of anecdotal evidence that having a colon irrigation done is good for a person. The greater the amount of anecdotal evidence, the greater the amount of scepticism by those who cling to the strict dogma of medical proof. These persons already have closed minds. But the anecdotal evidence means that it is stories observed within individuals as opposed to a study. So this means, for example, that Mary had a colon hydrotherapy treatment done and she felt great so she told her friend Suzy about how she felt. This is anecdotal. If Suzy goes to get a colon hydrotherapy treatment done and she feels great and then tells Carol, this again is just anecdotal. The greater the amount of anecdotal evidence there is means that there are a lot of people using the treatment or protocol. That's all it means.

There are risks of injury to the colon. This is something I do agree with. If someone is untrained in the administration of a colon irrigation treatment, they are at risk of puncturing the colon wall or tearing the anus. But this risk is no less than someone who engages in anal sexual stimulation. I would say that for a colon irrigation treatment to be effective and safe the person considering it must have a thorough knowledge of what is involved and why. Without this basic knowledge of the what and why, any activity will be inherently dangerous like driving a car, riding a bike, or doing a colon irrigation. If you are considering having one done, find a qualified and experienced professional.

The issue with electrolyte imbalance in the colon. The lower colon contains many different items in it. There is partially decomposing food matter. There are bacteria (good and bad) in the stool. There are salts formed from the acid generation and neutralization process in digestion. There is water. There is mucus coating the inner walls. If a person were to do a doctor-ordered purge before a colonoscopy, there would be the same electrolyte imbalance. This is how I view the situation. One cleanse, whether it is for your personal benefit or prior to a medical treatment, would not cause an electrolyte imbalance that the body could not fix within a couple of days. So this is perfectly fine. If a person is going to do a series of colon irrigation treatments, like every day, then effort must be made to restore the colon environment by working with someone who is qualified and proficient in restoring the gut balance.

The risk of dependency on the treatment issue. I do agree that there is a very small risk of becoming dependent on it, but this risk is no less than someone becoming dependent on medical chemical (drug) treatments for any condition within the body. People with a specific ailment who take an artificial treatment risk becoming dependent on that treatment as the body adapts. However, dependency is only a risk from repeated use and abuse of any protocol whether drug intervention or physical intervention. A person engaged in the occasional colon irrigation along with a sensible, holistic approach to eating and living, need not worry about becoming dependent on it.

The Best Way to Do It

The colon irrigation or colon hydrotherapy is the method that uses the most amount of water in cleansing the colon tube. This way would be effective in washing out a lot of the matter. There are factors which impact how much stuff comes out. Consider if you eat a diet of only processed foods, which make a sticky, gooey paste in your colon. The water may have to work harder to wash out this type of matter, especially as it hardens when water is removed by the large intestine. Now consider the stool when it has lots of carrot fibre, green vegetable fibres, and other plant-based fibre. It is easier for the water to sweep this matter away.

So for me personally, if I were to schedule a colon hydrotherapy session for next week, I would begin eating a diet of raw fruit and vegetables for the week prior to the treatment. This would allow my colon to have a high amount of plant-based material in there for easier removal with the water.

The treatments that I have had were an hour long and involved the use of a stomach massage during the treatment along with a heating pad on the stomach. In my treatment, they also use alternating warm and cold water to stimulate the colon to expand and contract. This can feel like a cramp and you can ask the person to use only one temperature water if that is better for you.

Some Interesting Things to Note

The concept of doing a colonic is easier to accept for a woman than for a man in my general observation. This is because some men may see the act of having a colonic treatment done as emasculating. While as a woman, I can sympathize with men for their feelings, as a medical professional, and a health educator, I can totally say that men need to get over it and understand the entire procedure. In understanding the Why behind the procedure, one can begin to see How it can be beneficial to the human body. As a mother, wife, or girlfriend, the job is to help your guy see the benefit while ensuring that his male ego is not bruised by this important treatment. Maybe have him in the room with you while you have your own treatment done to see that it is safe and okay. And it may take a while before a man will agree to try it, so be patient.

The Alternative to a Full Colonic

The alternative to a full colonic is what we do in the hospital for patients who come into the ER with severe constipation. That is called an enema. We sometimes administer a water enema to try to help soften the patient's stool in the lower part of the colon in order for it to come out. The bags contain about 1 to 1.5 litres of water and they really only soften a small section of the stool in the colon. If the patient has stool that is hardened higher up in the colon, then it will not be sufficiently softened and will be painful as the bowel tries to force it down the colon.

The enema in the hospital is a short-term solution to a long-term problem. You see, once the patient goes home, they don't think of doing an enema themselves. They are just told to drink more water and take more soluble fibre.

I don't recommend anyone do an enema at home unless they have done some type of training on how to properly and safely use an enema bag. With improper use, there is a risk of injuring the spincter muscle or puncturing the colon wall near to the anus. Care and caution must be exercised, but this can be a very safe procedure once a person is knowledgeable in how to properly execute it.

What Would I Do if I Were Severely Constipated?

First off, I would schedule an appointment to see a naturopath doctor where they also perform colon hydrotherapy treatments in the clinic. Why? Because I'd want to speak to the naturopath about natural, holistic options for softening my stools and strengthening my bowel function. Then I'd want to have a colon hydrotherapy treatment to unlock the hard stool.

Secondly, I'd want to do an enema at home on a periodic basic for a short term in order to help keep the stool soft. But this is only short term.

Lastly, I'd totally transform my diet to incorporate foods that don't become gummy and sticky inside the colon. This means eating a diet of mostly unprocessed and unrefined foods. Plus, of course, I would increase my water intake.

And what would I expect from this? I would expect to have regular, natural bowel movements within a short time because my expectation is that my body will begin to regulate itself once the blockage and the cause of the blockage has been removed.

Chapter Summary

In this chapter, we have looked at the concept of colon hydrotherapy. We have also looked at some of the benefits of it and some of the concerns with the treatment. I have highlighted how it might be applicable in the hospital setting as well as in a clinic setting.

Chapter References

[1] Huffington Post, UK
http://www.huffingtonpost.co.uk/2012/12/17/bowel-cancer-awareness-audit-concerns-health-symptoms_n_2314206.html

* * * * *

Digestion and Colon Health

Chapter 5

* * *

"During World War I, sailors aboard a German cruiser, Kronprinz Wilhelm, ate beef, ham, bacon, cheese, potatoes, canned vegetables, dried peas/beans, white bread, margarine, tea, coffee, sugar, condensed milk, cake, champagne and beer. The entire diet consisted of cooked and processed foods. After six months on this diet, the crew was experiencing shortness of breath, paralysis, atrophied muscles, enlarged hearts, constipation, anemia, and muscle and joint pains." - Raymond Francis, Never Be Sick Again.

"Eating is one of the major things we do in our lives. Many people have no training on eating and so they live to eat instead of eating what is necessary to live life well. A living to eat approach is essentially digging your grave with your fork." - Jenny Berkeley, RN, Certified Holistic Nutritionist, Health Educator

* * *

In order to look at a healthy bowel and proper colon function, we have to look at the entire system from end to end, that is, from mouth to rectum.

Mouth and Oesophagus

Let us begin by looking at the point of entry of food into the body, which is the mouth. Your mouth has teeth for fully grinding your food into a mushy substance. The food is mixed with saliva which is slightly alkaline. This mixture begins a pre-digestion process of the food. This food moves down the oesophagus which is coated with a thin mucus layer and is moist and elastic. If the food is not sufficiently masticated, it will cause an unpleasant sensation as it travels along the oesophagus. If for some reason the person is not producing enough saliva, then the food will be abrasive as it goes down to the stomach.

Thus it is important to ensure that all food is properly chewed and mixed with saliva at this initial stage. It is fundamentally important as the inputs affect the outputs.

Dr. Michael Schecter, a holistic health dentist in Toronto, who has written for my holistic lifestyle magazine, EternityWatch, talks about the saliva in the mouth being a good indication of a person's risk for gum disease, and infections, and even the risk of heart issues resulting from bacteria going to the heart from the mouth.

The saliva in the mouth should be a bit alkaline. He performs tests on his patients to determine the alkalinity or acidity of the saliva. If the saliva is slightly acidic, it means that the mouth is in a state which promotes the destruction of the teeth and promotes the growth of bacteria. It also means that the saliva is not effectively preparing food prior to it moving into the stomach.

This acidity is another tiny signal that a person must pay attention to as it is an indication of what is going on in their entire body. Remember, the body is a connected whole, not one piece in isolation. This speaks to the fundamental schools of thinking called reductionism and holism but that topic is another book.

For our purposes, we need to focus on making sure the saliva does its two main jobs. It has to begin to break down the food as it should and it needs to add sufficient moisture to the food to allow it to travel down to the stomach without causing discomfort along the way.

In order to ensure that the oesophagal tract is properly lubricated prior to eating, I would drink a cup or two of lukewarm water about 30 minutes prior to eating. I would drink this in slow mouthfuls that are swallowed and allowed to coat the lining as it travels. You should be able to feel the water. This is preparation for digestion.

Stomach

The stomach is a muscle that is designed to expand and contract as it mulches the masticated food. While this mulching is taking place, stomach acid is being mixed in with the food in order to break down larger food particles into a size that is readily absorbed in the small intestine.

The pH of the stomach must be very low, or another way to say it is the stomach must be very acidic. This acidity serves two purposes. First it further breaks down the food particles into more readily available forms. Secondly the acidity acts as a sterilization method for killing microbes that may have been in the food.

No liquid should be added into the stomach once it begins producing acid to lower the pH. If any liquid is added, this liquid raises the pH, or to put it another way, it makes the environment more alkaline and less acidic. When this happens two things will result.

Food will not be properly broken down in the stomach when the pH is raised too much. Bacteria and microbes that should have been killed by the stomach acid will escape to pass into the intestines where the risk of doing greater harm increases.

When you have this increased risk, you also risk greater infection and inflammation of the small intestines and/or the large intestines as the food moves along. To err on the side of caution, it is best to allow your stomach to do its job properly with stomach acid that is at the correct pH. So don't interfere with it by drinking during your meal.

The output from this step in the process is a soupy sludge that is highly acidic, which goes into the small intestine.

Small intestines

If the food has been processed properly in the stomach, a soupy, acidic sludge will be entering the small intestine. Here the body will neutralize this acidity by mixing it with the very alkaline bile fluids. From basic high school chemistry class you will understand that when an acid and alkaline are mixed together there is a neutralization, some salts produced, and/or even some gases.

The pH of the liquid food or sludge is raised to an alkaline state to allow it to travel through the small intestine without damaging the intestinal wall. This damage would be in the form of irritation of the mucus membranes and villi of the intestines. This irritation would then lead to inflammation, discomfort, and possible severe intestinal conditions. Of course, you want to avoid these things.

When the process works as it should, food nutrients are extracted from the solution as it passes through the small intestine. Food that is too big to be extracted is moved along towards the large intestines.

A risk of not chewing food well is that large portions may become lodged in the intestine or colon. This could lead to it rotting in there which increases risks to the health of the colon.

If you do not have sufficient water in your body prior to eating, then this solution of nutrients and food is thicker than it should be, causing it to move slower and/or coat the intestinal wall and inhibit absorption of nutrients in the future. Think of putty moving through a tube to give you an idea of what you want to avoid.

Large intestines

In the large intestine the focus is on the absorption of liquid from the nutrient solution. As the solution moves from the beginning of the large intestine towards the colon and rectum, it becomes harder and harder until it should leave the body as a soft, pasty stool.

There should be no pain or discomfort in this type of elimination and it should occur on a regular basis. A movement of two or three times per day for the average adult is well within a healthy range from a holistic health point of view.

The importance of following health rules of eating

Just as eating a healthy, nutritious meal is important for overall health, it is also important to eat your food in the correct time, in the correct manner, and following the correct rules for health and well-being.

Why many people mess up in this area is because the result of doing it wrong is not immediately apparent.

Let's look at something like baking. Suppose you had to bake bread at 400 degrees for 1 hour, but instead baked it at 250 degrees for that hour. At the 10-minute or 20-minute mark, you would not be able to tell that anything was wrong with your procedure.

It is only at the end of the hour when you removed the dough and examined it that you would be able to tell that the procedure was incorrect.

This is like our rules of eating today. Many people eat incorrectly and their wonderful bodies compensate a bit here and a bit there without them knowing the overall impact of the poor choice. Then after a few decades when the body can no longer compensate, they are hit with serious diseases.

So for the purpose of our look at colon health, we must focus on the general rules that will enable us to do our part to help our bodies maintain overall health and wellness.

Eating

Having outlined the major areas of the digestive system where the food will travel, we'll look at what is the best way we should eat.

The best way is a diet that is based on a whole foods, plant-based approach to eating. If you can eat raw, ripe, fresh, organic, and locally in season, then you will be giving your body what it needs from your particular region.

The book, Fresh Food4Life, part 4 of the Holistic Health Nurse Series of books, focuses more intently on the concept of eating and why we need to structure, or rather restructure, our eating habits for health and sustainability. If you want to learn more about the entire food supply structure and why we need to take action, pick up a copy of the book by clicking on the link, or visit Amazon.com to get it.

When to Eat

I follow and recommend a routine of three meals a day with no snacking in-between. However, the first meal of the day is always a liquid meal only. This could be a green smoothie or a green juice. It should be consumed early in the morning.

Lunch should follow four hours later. It is important to wait that long because you are allowing your stomach sufficient time to process the food and clean out the stomach. Then you are giving your stomach muscles a little bit of rest time before the next meal.

Supper time (or dinner time) should be four hours after you have completed your lunch meal and should not be a heavy meal. Suppose you start lunch at noon and finish at 1 p.m. Then your supper time would be at 5 p.m.

Now people may say, "I can't live like that, I'll feel too hungry" or "I'll feel tired," or any number of excuses. I'll suggest to you that the reason you feel this way is because of a "habit hunger" and not an actual need for food.

An ancient principle states, "eat for strength and not for gluttony." The eating times I have suggested here are sufficient for maintaining overall health and for rest times in between meals.

How much to eat

I cannot say that one person should eat a little bowl of rice or a soup and salad. If a person's stomach muscle has been stretched large, then it will take time for that person to feel full until their stomach has returned to a normal size.

So I do not have a one-size-fits-all approach here. But I have a great guideline. First begin with salad. Eat a big portion of that. The salad should be filled with fresh, living foods including sprouts like sunflower sprouts, radish sprouts, microgreens, and such.

Once you eat that big bowl of salad and have chewed the food properly, wait 60 to 120 seconds, quietly seated. If you still feel hungry, you can go ahead and consume a raw/living food gourmet dish if you are on a living foods diet, or a cooked vegan dish if you are eating cooked foods. It should be about 1/2 the size of the bowl of salad.

After you have finished eating your quantity of food, wait for another 60 to 120 seconds. Pay attention to your body signals. You should not be feeling hungry anymore. If you are still hungry, you can eat some carrots or cucumber and green leafy vegetables. The fibre in these vegetables will help you to feel full.

Do not eat until you feel like you want to burst. This is a sign that you have overeaten and your stomach muscle is stretched too much. Eat until you feel contented but not stuffed. Once you have reached that level, do not eat again for the next 4 hours. No dinner mints. No chewing gum. No

Tic-Tacs. Nothing more should go into your mouth except water which can only be consumed after a certain amount of time has passed. I discuss this in the chapter on water.

The Diet Components

This book, as with all of my books, promotes a plant-based diet because it is the diet that is sustainable for long-term health and wellness. Numerous studies have shown that a diet that is free of meat, dairy, and other animal products, leads to fewer cases of heart disease, diabetes, obesity, and other diseases.

My other books cover diet in detail. For the purpose of this book, I'll cover items beneficial for those focusing on colon health.

Plant-based fibre: This is something that is very desirable in your diet for your colon health. Plant-based fibre acts as a broom to sweep out the colon. Note that this fibre is from raw fruits or veggies, not cooked plant foods. However, lightly steamed plant foods are still acceptable. Some of my favourites include kale, spinach, celery, cabbage, cucumbers, carrots, lettuce and Swiss chard. These plant-based fibres can be used in salads, green smoothies, some raw-living food wraps, and even with dips. I strongly recommend a diet of 70% living foods for long-term health and vitality, including your colon health.

Fresh juices: Never again buy a juice from concentrate, from a tin, or in a packet. If you have to drink juice, make it yourself from the fresh fruit or vegetable. Buy an inexpensive juicer to get you started. And use it to make your fresh juice and drink it daily.

Supplements: When you are working on healing your digestive system, you may need to take a few supplements. These can be digestive supplements, probiotics, minerals, and enzymes. I discuss this in more detail in the chapter on that. However, know that you will need to add this into your diet at least in the short term.

<u>Water:</u> The type of water you drink is very important to your colon. The purpose of water is to hydrate your body and facilitate the proper function of every organ and cell in your body. Water is NOT juice, tea, coffee, or anything with added nutrients. Water is just water. And I have devoted an entire chapter on water in this book because it is vitally important to your colon health.

Chapter Summary

In this chapter we looked at the role of digestion in the goal of colon health. We did a walk-through of the different phases of the digestive cycle and looked at the input and output from one stage to the next. We also looked at eating. We looked at what to eat, when to eat, and the components of a diet designed for colon health.

* * * * *

Pay Attention to Your Body

Chapter 6

* * *

"I knew what my job was; it was to go out and meet the people and love them." - Diana, Princess of Wales

"To be attentive to your body and not dismissive of the little aches and pains and subtle signals, is to be closely aligned with knowing yourself and caring well for yourself." - Jenny Berkeley, RN, Certified Holistic Nutritionist, Health Educator

* * *

The sad thing about people in today's modern society is that they have become almost completely disconnected from their body needs on a natural level of understanding. This could be because of the tremendous amount of noise being generated by our digital world on a physical, electromagnetic, and mental level.

People have also been indoctrinated with a belief system that only mildly benefits them while benefiting those who would profit from the average person's lack of knowledge. Thankfully there are many health and wellness experts today, as well as conventional doctors and alternative doctors who wholeheartedly want to serve people and make our community a better place.

My focus on holistic health is because I am concerned about the coming pandemic of sickness facing Canadians. As the baby boomers are aging into their mid-60s and older, they are becoming sicker due to their lifestyle, the pollution of their environment, and their aging bodies' inability to heal faster. They will begin to place a tremendous burden on the medical system as they get sicker and sicker while doctors and nurses remain in short supply. Also my concern is for the children of the baby boomers who are in their mid-to-late 40s. Some of them are sandwiched between sick or mildly disabled parents and children who are sick or disabled. They themselves are in a terribly stressful situation, coping the best they can, but their life is making them sicker day by day. But they are under so much pressure that they cannot afford to get sick because their parents and children need them.

A while back, I saw a relatively young couple in the hospital, mid-to-late 40s or early 50s. I often try to bond with my patients as hospitals can be a cold place, especially when someone is ill. The husband was in the bed and was told that he would die within some months. The wife was heartbroken and weeping. I hugged her and I found myself crying also with her as I held her. They had young children and she was concerned about how she would be able to raise their children without their father, the man she loved with all her heart.

And there are many more times I have cried with my Canadian patients. Their story is not unique. Their pain and suffering, fear and sorrow, is one of many more that I see.

My heart is sore from all that crying. I want my fellow Canadians to take back control of their health where it is possible. Not every disease can be healed completely as every person's body and lifestyle is different. But everyone deserves the chance to try their best. No family needs to have to go through the worry of being broken up by a death of their loved one prematurely.

In contrast, we have the story of Linda Morin. She contributed an article in my holistic health magazine, EternityWatch Magazine. Her story was one of such courage — facing breast cancer and a double mastectomy. She was a single mother with two young boys.

She had her moments of fear, of tears, of sadness, and she had sacrificed part of her body. But her life experienced some moments that turned it around. She went on to publish a book about her life and her victory. Part of her victory in her emotional healing was a plant-based diet.

The reason you need to understand this

I don't want my readers to have cancer before they take notice. I don't want people to be sandwiched between sick children and sick parents feeling burnt out and trapped. I want people to feel in control and feel empowered.

That begins with knowledge. After living a life of ignorance of holistic health principles for health and wellness, it is time for those in their 30s and 40s to learn and implement sound health principles. Because the sick may need the healthy to provide care to them in a time of national emergency. Even if there is no emergency, as an individual, you need to be healthy for those around you who love and depend on you for support and guidance.

And so the reason you need to understand this is because there are others depending on you. And you need to be well yourself to fully add value to those around you.

The first step is quietness

The very first step on this journey is for you to find those hours of quietness in your day. There are 24 hours in a day. Eight of these hours will be spent in sleep. The other 16 will be spent on the daily activities of life. I'd like you to find just one hour out of the 16 for quietness and peaceful reflection. It could be 30 minutes in the morning and 30 minutes at night. This time is tremendously important to you and your journey on a holistic health lifestyle.

In this quiet time where you can meditate on your life and listen to your body, practice going deep within yourself and listening to your breathing, listening or feeling to your heart beat, feeling those tender joints, aching muscles, sore tummy, and more.

It may be very difficult, and in fact, could be one of the most challenging things you do each day considering your current lifestyle, but it is essential for you and your future to begin learning how to be sensitive to your body today.

Your body is communicating with you

Your body is not a dumb machine that you happen to inhabit. Even machines we use like cars have indicator lights which help us know what the car needs. There is a light when the car needs gas; there is a light when it needs oil; there is a light when it needs maintenance. But before the gas light, there is a gauge which allows you to see the gas level during your daily drive.

The body also has communication methods much like those gauges and lights. You can think of the indicator lights as when you get a serious disease which is not life threatening but forces you to stop and read and evaluate everything in your life. The gauges are the tiny aches, pains, soreness, stiffness, and other symptoms you experience during the course of the day or week and yet you ignore them in order to keep on going.

When the headache becomes too much, a person might pop a pill, typically an over-the-counter painkiller. Does this get to the root of the problem or simply numb the pain to allow you to proceed with your activity? The mild painkiller allows you to ignore your body signal, but this is not a good thing to do.

Imagine a car making a horrible noise under the hood and instead of taking it to a mechanic to find the problem, you turn on the radio louder to drown out the noise and continue driving. Does the loud music solve the problem of the noise under the hood? Of course not. Does the loud music allow you to drown out the sound to continue about your business? Yes, that is exactly what is happening. This is exactly what most people are doing with their bodies.

Small signals

If your body is communicating with you, what are some of those small signals that you should be looking for? There are so many that your body will give you for different things, but I have to limit my discussion to the digestive system and colon health.

Here's my own checklist for small signals not to be ignored:

1. Sluggishness when you have a bowel movement.
2. Feeling like there is still poop or feeling not satisfied after you poop.
3. Soreness in the stomach or lower abdominal region.
4. Bad breath.
5. Dry pellets in your stool.
6. Tiredness after eating.

These are the six signals you can experience from your body. If you are experiencing these things regularly, then you have to begin to reconsider what you are doing and listen to the body's cry for assistance.

Larger signals

Then there are larger signals that mean you need to really get your act together and start taking action to resolve the problem before your body breaks down:

1. Feeling of heartburn after a meal.
2. Mild constipation.
3. Feelings of thirst while eating or directly after eating.
4. Forcing or straining to defecate.
5. Allergies to foods previously not a problem.
6. Severe heartburn/acid reflux.

System Breakdown

When a person ignores the small signals and the larger signals, then all that is left for your body to do is to have a system breakdown. This is where you have the BIG diseases like chronic constipation, IBS, Crohn's Disease, Celiac, Colon Cancer and more.

In the later chapters we discuss a few of these dis-eases and some of the ways a person can approach them from a holistic point of view.

Remember that every body is different with different experiences, toxins, stresses, and being fed a different diet. So what works fast for one person may work slower for another. The important thing is to begin listening to your body and experiencing what is working and what is not. Then following up.

Is there hope?

For many people who are not in a system breakdown situation there is hope. I would say that for 95% of the people if they have the correct knowledge and are working with a qualified health and wellness professional to help them. For people in a system breakdown situation, I would say that there is a 50% chance of reversal for those who are not too far gone and are working with someone who is a professional in those types of cases.

Working with such professionals will take time and will cost money for the knowledge and expertise of those individuals. And in fact, I am very selective about who I work with because I am also busy with my many endeavours. I will only work with those people who fall within the range I can provide help and those who are willing to pay my fees. I also work with people who are willing to do what it takes. It does not make sense for me to take on a client otherwise.

If someone wants to get well for free, they can do two things. Pray to their god for help like their life depended on it AND get to the library and read every single book on their disease and a holistic approach to diet, lifestyle, living foods, and dealing with emotional stress. If a person has the time, and the determination, to do this, they may be able to find the answers that they need.

My book is a good first step and it is part of my Holistic Health Nurse Series of books on holistic health and wellness.

Find support on your journey

Along with listening to your body, seeking a qualified professional, and seeking knowledge yourself, you should find support from those closest to you. They could be your children, your spouse, your parents, or your siblings. If you have five brothers and sisters and two are supportive while three are negative, then ask the three to keep away and ask the two to stick closer.

This is important because you need all the love and support during any transition. The transition itself is hard enough without having to experience extra stress and negativity from those close to your heart.

Never give up

While you have life inside of you, you must always be hopeful and never give up. This is my ultimate message to all those who interact with me, read my books, articles, magazine, and my website. The human spirit is a power source that can fuel us to the good things we desire. But we must make the conscious decision to choose those things which are good for us.

My motto: "Good health is your birthright, Keeping it is your choice."

Choose well.

Chapter Summary

In this chapter we talked about your approach to health
from a personal point of view. This chapter emphasized the
need to listen to your body. It gives you signals long before
the situation gets bad. This is especially true where your
digestive system and colon are concerned.

If you want to have a healthy colon by design, you have to
be mindful of the signals and take corrective action as
needed. Like maintaining a car engine, if you maintain your
body, it will run well for you.

* * * * *

Magnesium and Colon Health

Chapter 7

* * *

"The man who will not execute his resolutions when they are fresh upon him can have no hope from them afterwards; they will be dissipated, lost and perished in the hurry and scurry of this world, or sunk in the slough of indolence." - Maria Edgeworth

"From my careful study of the material on Magnesium, I am convinced that it is a wonderful, necessary element for the body in its natural bio-available form." - Jenny Berkeley, RN, Health Educator

* * *

Magnesium is one of the most important elements needed in the human body. According to internationally known medical doctor and naturopathic doctor, Dr. Carolyn Dean, magnesium is one of the greatest things that you can ingest to help your body. She has written extensively on the topic of magnesium and has devoted a large part of her professional work to the study of magnesium.

In this chapter I will be covering some of the reasons you need to ensure that you have enough magnesium in your body to support your overall health and wellness, and your digestive health.

Magnesium is a co-factor for over 325 enzymes that execute vital metabolic functions in the human body. Magnesium can greatly help with numerous lifestyle diseases and chronic diseases, however it is not a first option that is used within the medical profession.

What is magnesium?

Magnesium is, in layman's terms, a sister element of iron. What I mean to say is that, as iron is to the blood of human beings, magnesium is to the chlorophyll (blood) of plants. In our human blood, iron forms the central element of haemoglobin. It is the cornerstone upon which the haemoglobin blood cell is built. If there is no iron or little iron in the body, then the body will not produce sufficient red blood cells. Magnesium is a similar functioning element in the production of chlorophyll in plants. It is this chlorophyll in the plants that helps them convert the sun's energy into their plant cells, leaves, shoots, and fruit. And given the significance of magnesium in the plant world, it is understandable that as humans need plant-based foods for survival, magnesium is an important part of that equation.

How is magnesium delivered into the human body?

There are several ways that magnesium can find itself inside the human body. First you can get magnesium by eating a wide variety of leafy green vegetables, consuming wheat grass juice or other grass juices, taking magnesium-based supplements, and drinking a fully mineralized water source like water from a spring. And of course with each way of consuming magnesium there are a variety of costs associated with it. Water could be considered the cheapest if you live near a well or natural spring, while purchasing supplements would be considered the most expensive.

Signs That You Could Be Magnesium Deficient

According to the research of Dr. Carolyn Dean, she has found these factors that tend to indicate a person might be deficient in magnesium.

1. Alcohol intake - more than seven drinks per week.
2. Anger
3. Angina
4. Anxiety

5. Apathy
6. Arrhythmia of the heart
7. Asthma
8. Blood work showing:
   a) low calcium   b) low potassium   c) low magnesium
9. Bowel problems
   a) Undigested fat in the stool
   b) constipation
   c) diarrhoea
   d) alternating constipation and diarrhoea
   e) IBS
   f) Crohn's disease
   g) Ulcerative Colitis
10. Brain trauma
11. Bronchitis, chronic
12. Caffeine intake
13. Chronic fatigue syndrome
14. Cold extremities
15. Concentration difficulties
16. Confusion
17. Convulsions
18. Depression
19. Diabetes (a. Type I   b. Type II   c. Gestational diabetes)
20. Fibromyalgia
21. Food intake imbalances
a. Limited in green leafy vegetables, seeds, and fresh fruit
b. High protein
22. Food cravings
a. Carbohydrates
b. Chocolate
c. Salt
d. Junk food
23. Gagging or choking on food
24. Hand Tremor
25. Headaches
26. Heart disease
27. Heart - rapid rate
28. High blood pressure
29. Homocystinuria
30. Hyperactivity

31. Hyperventilation
32. Infertility
33. Insomnia
34. Irritability
35. Kidney stones
36. Medications
a. Digitalis
b. Diuretics
c. Antibiotics
d. Steroids
e. Oral contraceptives
f. Indomethacin
g. Cisplatin
h. Amphotericin B
i. Cholestyramine
j. Synthetic estrogens
37. Memory impairment
38. Mercury amalgam dental fillings
39. Menstrual pain and cramps
40. Migraines
41. Mineral supplements
a. Take calcium without magnesium
b. Take zinc without magnesium
c. Take iron without magnesium
42. Mitral valve prolapse
43. Muscle cramps or spasms
44. Muscle twitching or tics
45. Muscle weakness
46. Numbness of hands or feet
47. Osteoporosis
48. Paranoia
49. Parathyroid hyperactivity
50. PMS
51. Polycystic ovarian disease
52. Pregnancy
a. Currently pregnant
b. Pregnant within one year
c. History of preeclampsia or eclampsia
d. Postpartum depression
e. Have a child with cerebral palsy

53. Radiation therapy, recent
54. Raynaud's syndrome
55. Restlessness
56. Sexual energy diminished
57. Shortness of breath
58. Smoking
59. Startled easily by noise
60. Stressful life or circumstances
61. Stroke
62. Sugar, high intake daily
63. Syndrome X
64. Thyroid hyperactivity
65. Tingling of hands or feet
66. Transplants
a. Kidney
b. Liver
67. Water that contains the following
a. Fluoride
b. Chlorine
c. Calcium
68. Wheezing

Magnesium and Your Digestive Health

How is magnesium important to our discussion on digestive health? Well, the obvious ways are the disease outline above based on Dr. Carolyn Dean's work and research. The diseases of interest to us include:

The Bowel dis-eases: These are the occurrences of the undigested fats in the stool, the frequent constipation, the diarrhoea, the alternating constipation and diarrhoea, the IBS, the Crohn's disease, and the Ulcerative Colitis. These are the diseases of the lower part of the digestive system that we want to consider in regards to magnesium.

The Upper Digestive Tract dis-eases: These would be the gagging or choking on food, the food cravings for junk food, excessive acidity in the mouth and saliva, and the acid reflux condition.

Now I'm not going to tell you that magnesium will cure all these conditions. The human body is tremendously complex and removing a symptom of dis-ease takes a holistic approach and effort. However Dr. Carolyn does offer some promising hope where magnesium is concerned.

Let me tell you how magnesium works in the body and with this knowledge you may be able to see how magnesium can influence your particular condition.

Magnesium Aids in Acid/Alkaline Balancing

On a daily basis and as a result of the thousands of biological and enzymatic processes which take place in your body, your body creates a substantial amount of acid waste. It is this acidic waste which over time reduces your body's ability to function at optimal level.

Magnesium is an alkalizing mineral. Within the body, magnesium along with calcium, can be used to neutralize the various points of acidity whether at a cellular level or within the digestive system or as the result of metabolic processes. Thus when you are ensuring that you have a sufficient amount of magnesium within your biological system, i.e., your body, you give your body another tool in fighting over acidity.

From a digestive system perspective, magnesium could be helpful with the body's regulation of the pH of the saliva, the mouth, and the mucus lining leading to the stomach.

As the acid sludge exits the stomach into the small intestines, the body may be able to quickly turn the pH back into an alkaline state where nutrients can be absorbed.

Magnesium and muscle tissue

Magnesium works within the body to relax muscle cells while calcium causes muscle cells to contract. The ability of magnesium to cause muscle tissue to relax regardless of where it is located within the body means that sore and aching muscles can relax with the application of magnesium. Magnesium is also used to neutralize the buildup of lactic acid in muscle tissue and it is depleted as a result of sweating during exercise.

Now consider the digestive tract from the mouth to the stomach. It is a fleshy, muscular tube that expands and contracts to move the food down from the mouth to the stomach. If you are having difficulty in this region of the digestive tract, it could be that the muscle is deficient in the relaxing power of magnesium.

The stomach is also a muscle. It contracts and expands as it goes about the work of mulching the semi-solid food and converting it into a liquid sludge. The stomach muscle also needs to ensure that it maintains sufficient flexibility and elasticity when it expands and contracts. Magnesium may also be beneficial in this regard.

Now the lower part of the digestive system consisting of the small intestines, large intestines, and colon, are also muscular tissues that expand and contract in what is called peristalsis in order to move the food towards your anus. Knowing what we know about the relaxing power of magnesium on muscle tissue, we can surmise that sufficient intake of magnesium may be beneficial in helping this muscle to assume relaxation after a contraction and aid in maintaining proper elasticity of the muscle tissue.

Dr. Carolyn notes, "If muscles are deficient in magnesium, they become irritated and on edge developing tics, twitches, and outright spasms." This could explain why some people develop stomach cramps in some cases, and/or even part of a spastic colon. When the body has optimum levels of magnesium, the cells are relaxed and there is a natural calm throughout the entire body system.

Magnesium and water retention

Magnesium is one of the most important minerals you need to help maintain the water content in your colon. The doctors will tell you that you need a lot of fibre in order to assist with proper bowel movements. This is true, but you also need a lot of moisture to move the soupy sludge across the intestines. If your food waste remains in the colon for too long, your body will continuously keep removing the water from it. This will result in its hardening until it becomes almost like rocks or pellets. At this stage you should recognize that this is not a healthy situation. By ensuring you have sufficient magnesium in your food waste, it will act as a magnet to hold the moisture content longer in your colon until you have eliminated the waste.

For example, if you are going on a long journey where it may be difficult to find a toilet to eliminate your stool, then you may find that your stool will be hard when you eventually use the toilet. In order to counteract this problem you might want to take a small amount of magnesium supplement 24 to 48 hours before the trip so that there will be sufficient magnesium in your colon to allow for the stool to stay soft for the duration of the trip.

If you find that you frequently have hard stool, then perhaps you are experiencing a deficiency in magnesium in your body and thus your colon is not retaining water as well as it should. Typically an over-the-counter magnesium supplement should be sufficient to help in the short term only.

Ultimately you will need to build up your body's magnesium stores by consuming a diet of foods which are rich in magnesium. And it may take several months before your body is able to build up sufficient reserves, but once that has happened you should notice a change in the moisture content and regularity of your bowel elimination.

Magnesium and Detoxification

Magnesium is also a wonderfully important mineral for the removal of toxic substances, heavy metals such as aluminium and lead, and excess minerals like calcium from the human body.

Magnesium is the fundamental component of chlorophyll. When you ingest chlorophyll in the form of your green juices and green leafy vegetables, you are getting an incredibly remarkable chelating agent. What do I mean by that? The chelating agent is one that binds with other substances in the body to make it inert and readily available for excretion by the body. This means that the body is able to detoxify itself of the unwanted substance with less energy and greater efficiency.

Let's take a hypothetical example to simply illustrate this point. Suppose you had a toxin called aluminium inside your body. And suppose this aluminium had found a way to bind with certain key points along your spine. This electromagnetic bond would be so strong that the body itself would have great difficulty breaking the bond and eliminating the aluminium. Now when the magnesium-rich chlorophyll goes into the body and goes near to the site of the aluminium bond, the chlorophyll binds more strongly to the aluminium causing it to release its hold in your body. The electromagnetic bond created inside the aluminium-chlorophyll is so strong that the aluminium will not bind to anything else in the body. And your body will eliminate this compound safely.

As we look at this from the perspective of a healthy digestive system, we can see that having sufficient magnesium/chlorophyll in your digestive tract can bind/chelate with harmful toxins before they even enter the bloodstream and cause damage. Thus they may be safely eliminated in the stool.

Are you lacking magnesium?

Magnesium is essential from the womb. If your mother was not ensuring that her magnesium reserves were high enough, it would have impacted both you and her during those formative months.

While I cannot stress enough how important magnesium is to the human body and to a holistic approach to health, I must also say that in today's society getting enough magnesium in your daily diet is not as easy as it was 100 or 150 years ago.

For example, let's look at the soil. One hundred and fifty years ago the soil quality and water quality across the globe was good. Farmers could still grow the crops and produce derived from those plants were loaded with essential nutrients and phyto-nutrients.

Now we have a situation where crops are planted in soil that is suffering from chronic mineral deficiency. This is due to decades of mono-cropping which has caused many of the nutrients to be depleted from the soil. So when we buy fruits and vegetables today, we are actually getting fruits and vegetables that contain less mineral density than crops from more than one hundred years ago. Plus crops have been bred to produce more sweetness now than long ago.

Another thing is that "fresh" produce is picked green before the plant has had sufficient time to extract more minerals from the soil and deposit them into the cell structure of the fruits and veggies. Then the fruit is ripened on the boat, train, and truck ride. To give you a simple illustration, let's suppose a fully ripe mango, picked just as it falls from the tree, contains 300mg of magnesium. But if this mango is picked green in order to ship to another country, it may only have 100mg of magnesium. Even as it ripens in-transit, it still only contains 100mg of magnesium because it is no longer connected to the source of nutrients from the earth. And though it looks as perfectly ripe and juicy as the same mango that would fall from the tree, it only contains a portion of the nutrients.

Now consider that this is the same type of scenario for all produce picked green and shipped to another country for consumption. Unless you are growing your own crops in a rich medium, you are getting fewer nutrients than you should from your diet. Thus you are losing access to one vital level of access to magnesium.

You are also losing magnesium from poor diet and lifestyle choices today.

Steps to rebuilding your magnesium reserves

There are two ways to get magnesium into your body. One method is via the use of synthetic magnesium substances. The second method is via the use of plant-based, whole food, bio-available magnesium.

These are two very similar yet very different ways of getting magnesium in your body. The simple way I can explain it is like the difference between a dead almond and a living almond. If you put both seeds in the ground, nature will prove to you which one brings forth life.

With the synthetic magnesium, even thought it may be a compound that is similar to the bio-available counterpart, it is an isolate and therefore only marginally effective on your body. Magnesium oxide is one example. It is only slightly absorbed in the intestinal tract and instead goes right through the body. Thus it has more of a laxative purpose than a supplemental proper.

Magnesium oil is another method of getting magnesium. It is used externally. By rubbing this on the skin, it is absorbed. It does not produce a laxative effect that one will experience when taking synthetic magnesium orally.

The other way to get magnesium is via your whole-food supplements or simply by eating more foods that contain a higher magnesium content.

Magnesium Content of Common Foods (The Magnesium Miracle pg. 230)

Food	Magnesium mg/100g serving
Kelp	760
Wheat bran	490
Wheat germ	336
Almonds	270
Cashews	267
Buckwheat	229
Dulse	220
Millet	162

I would also add more green juices with lots of chlorophyll into my daily routine. I personally love juices that are made from kale, spinach, wheatgrass, Swiss chard, and other greens.

Chapter Summary

In this chapter we have looked at the importance of magnesium as it pertains to your digestive health. We have gone through an overview of magnesium and how it works inside of the digestive tract. We have also looked at ways to add magnesium back into your diet and replenish your body's resources.

Chapter References

How To Change Your Life With Magnesium
The Magnesium Miracle

* * * * *

Supplements and Digestive Health

Chapter 8

* * *

"Genetics may load the gun, but environment pulls the trigger." - Pamela Peeke, M.D., M.P.H.

"Sometimes a person who has lived a specific way has used up some of the important nutrients their body needs. At these times supplements are needed to boost up the body's supply while the person is restructuring their lives around a wholesome, healthy diet." - Jenny Berkeley, RN, Certified Holistic Nutritionist, Health Educator

* * *

On a cellular level, we can consider the onset of disease a fundamental breakdown of the cells' ability to fight off that which makes them sick. Cells are created to live for their purpose, and then die. They also reproduce healthier cells or sicker cells depending on the environment which they are a part of.

In the context of digestive and colon health, we want to have cells in that region that are functioning according to their purpose and we want them to produce healthier cells after them. Supplements can help by changing the influences in the environment around the cells.

What are supplements?

In general terms, supplements are items we consume in order to raise our intake level of specific nutrients, combat deficiencies, or stimulate cleansing. By making use of supplements, you are actively participating in redesigning the environment of your colon.

Probiotics

Trillions of microorganisms live in your intestinal tract. You have two sides constantly battling for dominion of your intestines. The good bacteria, also known as probiotics, are on your side and help promote good health. The bad bacteria are the ones that if left unchecked, can cause you to experience a wide range of intestinal dis-eases.

Both the good and the bad intestinal flora are needed to do their job. When the digestive system is operating at optimal levels, there will be more beneficial bacteria than the bad. What you eat at any given meal influences the environment of your intestines and either helps your good guys or helps your bad guys.

If you have undergone any antibiotic regimen, then your intestinal flora could be out of whack. If you have been eating a diet which promotes the overgrowth of bad bacteria, then you need to take action to alter the terrain and restore balance.

Experts on the subject say that you should have a ratio of 85% good bacteria and 15% bad bacteria. It is not possible to manually check your ratio daily, but take it as a given that the majority of people have their gut flora out of whack. This can be from young children to mature adults and even seniors.

Why do you want to supplement with probiotics? You want to because they can be helpful with the following:
- Helping in digestion
- Helping in absorption of nutrients
- Helping with skin conditions
- Helping to fight yeast and fungal infections (including candida)
- Helping to keep other bad pathogens under control
- Helping to maintain correct pH
- Helping to regulate your bowel

The unfriendly bacteria like your colon to be in a toxic state. They create waste products that add to the toxic environment, making the place more hospitable to them and less hospitable to the good bacteria.

When you take a good probiotic, you are adding more reinforcements to the good guys in your intestines. Thus your actions can help tip the scale in their favour. Probiotics hinder the bad guys in your gut by the production of antibacterial substances which hinders the growth of the bad bacteria.

Prebiotics

You may not have heard of prebiotics. The simple way to explain it is, they are the food that the probiotics eat. There are many millions of good bacteria in the gut that need to be given the proper food for their function. These prebiotics are the proper food for helping your probiotics. These prebiotics are soluble fibres (carbohydrates) that stimulate the growth and activity of one or more beneficial gut bacteria.

These types of fibres are present in whole foods such as vegetables, fruits, whole grains, and legumes. These fibres feed the Bifidobacterium species.

Here are some traits of a good prebiotic:
- They are not digested or absorbed in the stomach.
- They produce a beneficial systemic effect on colon health.
- They can modify the bacteria flora in the gut, promoting balance.
- They promote growth of the friendly bacteria.

The soluble fibres meeting these are the oligosaccharides. Prebiotic supplements are most often made using fructooligosaccharides or inulins.

Some food sources of oligosaccharides include garlic, leeks, whole grains, barley, artichokes, dandelion greens, beans and legumes, and Jerusalem artichokes.

I love using all those foods and I even have organic Jerusalem artichoke growing in my backyard garden. I harvest them in the year and juice them with my vegetable juicer or lightly sauté them with some other veggies.

Digestive Enzymes

The digestive enzymes help our bodies to digest food substances. There are three main food types that our bodies use the enzymes to digest. The enzymes which digest proteins are called proteases. The enzymes which digest carbohydrates are called amylases. The enzymes which digest fats are called lipases.

These digestive enzymes are important for your overall health and your digestive health. They become even more important for a person eating a diet that is too rich with processed foods. Digestive enzymes work in cooperation with probiotics and help break down food and facilitate absorption of nutrients from the food.

A health routine of taking digestive enzymes can help a person with their overall digestive health. However, it is important to find one that is not a synthetic but rather a whole food-based supplement. There are also concerns that some digestive enzymes are derived from animals so vegans need to find a vegan option.

Your body produces these digestive enzymes, which are essentially proteins with charged bio-electrical activity. When a person is a child or teen, their bodies are able to produce enzymes to keep up with their digestive demand. However, when a person reaches 40, the body's ability to produce the needed enzymes decreases and the lower output has significant impact on colon health, digestive health, and overall health.

A poor diet while growing up naturally compounds the "burnout" of the body by the time a person reaches their forties. Thus, a good digestive enzyme supplement used periodically while growing up combined with a wholesome and healthful diet is important. But it is not too late to alter your diet.

Food Enzymes

This brings me to food enzymes. They are the enzymes found in your raw living foods. They are in fruits, vegetables, greens, root vegetables, etc. When you eat your food raw, that is, living food, you maintain and consume the food enzymes that will help to break down the food inside your digestive system.

The more naturally occurring enzymes in the food to facilitate its breakdown means the fewer supplements you need to take and the less work by your body to produce a lot of those digestive enzymes to break down your food.

This is one of the best reasons to move to a diet that is high in living foods and low in processed "dead" foods. Dr. Leonard Caldwell, one of the world's foremost cancer specialists recommends a diet of 70% raw, living foods.

This diet has been proven to be one that is consistent with overall health, wellness, and vitality. It is loaded with the food enzymes needed to break the food down and get those nutrients and phytonutrients into your body and feeding your cells.

Let's frame this in the context of colon health and digestive health. Within your gut, you need enzymes to help break down your food. You also need to intake prebiotics which are soluble fibre that helps to feed your friendly bacteria in your colon.

Raw foods contain all the plant-based fibres intact. They contain the living enzymes of the plant which help digest it within the body. They contain some pre-digested food nutrients that make it less work for your body to digest. Lastly, they contain insoluble fibre which acts as a broom to sweep out your intestines and your colon and move the toxic waste out.

Systemic Enzymes

Systemic enzymes are enzymes which are found throughout the body and help your body to function and carry out the activities of life. These systemic/metabolic enzymes work in many ways from items such as regulating biological functions, reducing inflammation, digesting scar tissue, boosting the immune system, facilitating the exchange of air in the lungs, keeping the blood clean, and much more.

Digestive enzymes work in the digestive system. Systemic enzymes, on the other hand, need to be all around the body. Thus systemic enzymes are taken on an empty stomach unlike digestive enzymes.

If you have inflammation in your intestines, then adding some systemic enzymes to your diet can help lessen the impact while your body is coping. It is always wise to work with a professional experienced in working with enzymes.

Next Steps

Over the years I have tried many different kinds of probiotics and supplements. Some were awful and made me feel sick, and some were derived from animals. Now I know better than to use an animal-based probiotic. You can find a good naturopathic doctor to work with you to set up a good regime. There should be no need to take an animal-based supplement or a synthetic supplement or isolate. If the person you are working with keeps trying to push you in that direction, then find someone else with the knowledge and skill to help you.

Chapter Summary

In this chapter I have tried to give you an overview of why supplements are important to your digestive health and colon health, and we focused more specifically on the enzymes and probiotics. A proper approach to colon health must take into account the importance of supplementation to rebuild and maintain health.

* * * * *

GMOs and Digestive Health

Chapter 9

* * *

"Physical courage, which despises all danger, will make a man brave in one way; and moral courage, which despises all opinion, will make a man brave in another. The former would seem most necessary for the camp; the latter for the council; but to constitute a great man, both are necessary." - Charles Caleb Colton.

"It is important for people to always look to the "why" concerning their health and the world that influences them. Genetically modified foods contain too many "whys" but not enough solid answers for the benefit of mankind. Thus, society should use the precautionary principle and individuals should not eat genetically modified foods." - Jenny Berkeley, RN, CHN, Health Educator

* * *

The issue of genetically modified organisms (GMOs) is one of utmost importance to the health and wellbeing of every person on the planet today. And it is not just every human today, but the health and wellbeing of our children and grandchildren that are at stake in this.

The consumption of GMOs has the potential to substantially negatively impact the proper functioning of your colon and your entire digestive system. It can throw things quite literally out of whack.

What are GMOs?

Genetically modified organisms are man-made organisms that are neither natural nor evolutionary. They are basically Frankenstein-monster organisms. Using scientific methods, big-agriculture-business scientists have been able to combine genes from multiple organisms that would never be able to mate in nature. Genetically modified organisms can be plants or animals.

What are some examples of GMOs?

Spider-goat[1]: Scientists have taken the DNA of a spider and mixed it with the DNA of a goat in order to get the goat to produce the spider web protein in its milk. The scientists want to use that spider-goat milk to create bulletproof vests and clothing.

Glo-Fish[1]: Scientists have taken the DNA of a jellyfish and inserted it into a zebrafish. They did this to make the fish glow. This fish is meant to be a pet for recreational/entertainment purposes. It was introduced to the U.S. market in December 2003 by Yorktown Technologies of Austin, Texas.

Fern-Spider[1]: The fern spider is another impossible creature in nature. Scientists have created a cross between a fern and a spider. The spider is an animal with ferns growing out of its body. This spider was genetically created to "test" the survival rate of the GMO spider.

Food Examples of GMOs

Genetically modified (or genetically engineered) foods are found in canola (rape seed), corn, soy, and sugar beets (white sugar beet for making sugar) which are grown in Canada. Canada imports crops which include GE papaya, GE squash, GE cottonseed oil, and milk products made with Bovine Growth Hormone.[2]

If we look at the five items: canola, corn, soy, sugar beets, and milk products, you can see the entire food supply can become contaminated with GE derived ingredients.

Consider canola, which is used to make canola oil. This cheap oil is used by individuals at home as well as in restaurants to prepare food items. Food is cooked in this GM oil and this is contaminated with the GMO.

Let's look at sugar beet, which is used to make white sugar. Sugar is used in drinks such as coffees, teas, and juices. If you go into a Tim Horton's or Starbucks, can you be 100% certain that the sugar packet or sugar cube is 100% GE free? It is more than likely that you are consuming GE sugar. Sugar is also used in bread-making to activate the yeast. Do you eat bread? Your bread could be contaminated with GE ingredients also.

Let's also consider corn. Corn is used to make corn flour, corn chips, and many other corn products including high fructose corn syrup (HFCS). This HFCS is a super sweetener added to commercial production of drinks like Coca-Cola, Pepsi, and other sugary sodas and pops. It is used in some of the larger food manufacturing processes because it is a cheap sweetener. In my research, I have even found that the sugar solution used to test pregnant mothers for gestational diabetes is derived from non-organic (read GMO) corn. This stunned me. This means that even if a mother eats organic for the benefit of her health and her unborn child's health, by taking the gestational diabetes test with the GMO sugar solution, she would be introducing the GMO contaminant into her system and that of her unborn child. Thankfully a mother who eats a healthy organic diet and has advanced knowledge of health principles can refuse to have that invasive test done on her unborn child, especially with the risk of GMOs.

GMO and Earth Impact

The impact of the genetically modified organisms to the earth are as yet unexplained. One thing is clear, however. In the plant world, there is no such thing as co-existence between GE crops and nature-made crops. Many farmers have found that pollen from the GE crops end up contaminating non-GE crops and so the resulting seed is contaminated forever. There is no way to undo the pollination once the genes have mixed.

GE crops are designed with the purpose of being resistant to chemical herbicides or capable of producing their own insecticide. These two features of the GE crops make them a cash cow for the herbicide manufacturers that also own the seed companies that produce the GE seed. One example of an herbicide-tolerant crop is the Roundup Ready soy and Bt corn made by Monsanto. Initially, the usage of herbicides decreased, but as farmers overused the chemical, the tolerance of the weeds around it grew. Thus more and more needed to be applied after a few years. According to one report[3],

"HT crops have increased herbicide use by 527 million pounds over the 16-year period (1996-2011). The incremental increase per year has grown steadily from 1.5 million pounds in 1999, to 18 million five years later in 2003, and 79 million pounds in 2009. In 2011, about 90 million more pounds of herbicides were applied than likely in the absence of HT, or about 24% of total herbicide use on the three crops in 2011."

This amounts to soaking the earth in toxic pesticide and herbicides. These toxic and poisonous (to certain plants, insects, and small animals) chemicals get into the water, into the environment, and eventually into us. Consequently, there are now over two dozen weeds that are resistant to glyphosate, the major ingredient in the Roundup pesticide.

All of the negative impacts of the GE crops have a ripple effect in our world. And most importantly, an impact on you.

GMOs are a definite threat to your colon health and digestive health

We mentioned glyphosate earlier but this is where one of the real threats to your body's homoeostasis exists. Glyphosate was originally patented as a chelating agent. This means that it binds with certain nutrients so tightly that nothing else can make use of those nutrients. When glyphosate is sprayed on weeds, it chelates or binds with nutrients that the plant needs. As the weed does not have access to those nutrients, it gets sicker and dies from plant diseases or insects. This is how glyphosate works on weeds.

The Roundup Ready crops are designed to be stronger than the chelating effect of the glyphosate so they do not die immediately. But since glyphosate only knows how to chelate, those crops sprayed with it are naturally lower in those trace minerals and vital minerals necessary for optimum health.

The crop then gets harvested and it goes in two directions. Some goes to humans to eat and some goes to animals to eat. The animals that eat the glyphosate-laden grass, or corn, or hay, will naturally end up lacking nutrients vital for optimum health. This is because the residual glyphosate on the crop leaves, stems, and fruit, are going to be eaten by the animal. Then glyphosate will do its job. It will chelate with the nutrients in the cattle or pig or sheep or any domesticated farm animal. And over time the animal will lack those nutrients that killed the weeds. The animals may not die immediately, but on all levels, the animal will get weaker. And any humans who eat these weakened animals which are more susceptible to diseases, thus are at greater risk of GE contamination and also disease contamination.

The crop that gets sent for human consumption makes it into processed food products such as flours, cereals, breads, etc. And the residual glyphosate on the processed crop ends up in your food and when you eat it, it chelates (binds) to essential nutrients in your body. It may not kill you immediately, but it will weaken your body from the inside out until you are overwhelmed by disease.

Issue #1: Glyphosate chelates/binds with the nutrients in your food and in your body, causing you to lose access to key nutrients for optimal health. Thus it makes your digestive process ineffective at getting you the nutrients you need.

The other problem with GE crops is the ones that naturally produce insecticides. In nature-made corn and cotton, those plants do not naturally produce a toxin to kill small insects. With the man-made GE corn and cotton, man has figured out a way to add a gene into those plants that causes the entire plant to produce trace amounts of the Bt toxin. This toxin works to kill insects by causing their stomachs to burst open when they eat the plant.

In India, where Bt cotton has been planted and where many farmers have committed suicide due to the use of GMO crops, they found that the GE cotton killed their small domestic animals such as the goats they raised.[4]

In other parts of the world, farmers have been intimidated, threatened, sued, and bullied by the corporate giant Monsanto when any negative comments or statements have been made about the GM crop. Some farmers lived in fear and would not speak on camera for a documentary, David versus Monsanto. In it you can see the stories of a couple of farmers who were brave enough to go on record with their personal stories of harassment and intimidation. Farmers have been made sick with stress from the ordeal, no doubt. Has this driven some farmers to quit being farmers? No one has asked this question for North America.

Issue #2: The GM crops are physically dangerous to farmers because of the increasing toxicity of the crops and the added pesticides. The GM crops are psychologically dangerous to farmers because of the bullying, harassment, and blatant disregard for their livelihood. GMOs and the business executives are a threat to farming and thus societies because if no one farms, there will be no food.

The third and most compelling reason to be aware of GMOs is the recent announcement by the American Food and Drug Administration agency that it has approved the GMO Salmon for use in the human food supply. That means they intend to allow it to be used for food. Even though the FDA had completed its EIA (Environment Impact Study) in May, it did not release this or its recommendation until December 21. Perhaps it had something to do with the Prop 37 campaign and the elections as this would surely have been a question posed to the presidential candidates. Nevertheless, the FDA recommendation will not go unchallenged by those in the real health movement.

Although it was completed by mid-May, being controversial in nature, it is no surprise that the FDA quietly released its Environmental Impact Assessment and recommendation that AquaBounty's GE salmon be approved on December 21st, well after the election and during the winter break. However, it did not work; numerous groups and individuals are rallying to prevent the FDA approval during the current 60-day comment period, which lasts until February 25th. It's interesting to note that approval to grow GMO salmon came from the FDA in 2010 according to CBC Canada[6].

Back in the summer of 2012 I wrote an article for the Hippocrates Health Institute magazine on the topic of GMO salmon and the long-term negative implications of it on our planet. In the article, I drew the linkage between consuming GMO plants and the genetic material transference to animals. This was shown in a study to test whether hens fed GMO feed could be considered GMO FREE. They could not as it was found that there was genetic material transference.

The findings are particularly powerful because the work was carried out by independent experts, rather than GM critics.

Now I simply ask you to consider the health risk of salmon; the risk of GM material transference to sea creatures such as predators of salmon, or smaller fishes is higher. Big fish eat little fish.

And this can come back to humans when they eat the salmon or any animal that ate the salmon. And the risk of contamination of the gut bacteria from multiple sources is indeed very high. There is also a GM bacteria that is used to create vitamin D used in some vitamin supplements.

Issue #3: The risk of contamination of your gut as well as transference of genetic material from GMO cellular material to your own human cellular material is a high risk that must be avoided.

The final threat I want to bring to your attention is based on a study in late 2012 which found that GMO foods transferred a toxic gene to humans.

It was led by Nancy Podevin, who was employed by EFSA, and Patrick du Jardin, of the Plant Biology Unit at the University of Liege in Belgium.

They discovered that 54 of the 86 GM plants approved for commercial growing and food in the U.S., including corn and soya, contain the viral gene, which is known as 'Gene VI'.

This Gene VI is another reason you need to be mindful of the dangers of consuming the genetically modified foods. Much of the dangers of all GMO crops and foods derived from those crops are still to be determined because there are no labels in North America to distinguish which people got sick from eating GMOs for 5 or 10 years. In Europe, where they require GMO labelling, there is a better chance to study people who eat GM foods knowing that it is labelled as such.

One concern with Gene VI is that it leads to overproduction of certain proteins in cells. The impact of this protein could be toxic, trigger allergic responses, or cause some other harmful impact.

In the movie, Genetic Roulette, Jeffrey Smith mentions a mysterious gene that attacks and kills the unborn fetus in any animals that consume a specific GMO food that contains the gene. One scientist explained how they determined that the gene was causing the miscarriages. First, they observed this weird condition in the animal. Then they isolated the gene. They grew the gene in a lab. They reintroduced the gene to the pregnant animal. They observed the same result. Then they isolated the gene again. This was then identified as the reason the farm animals losing their unborn babies.

Just think for a moment. If animals are losing their unborn to miscarriages, is it possible that the same gene could be causing a similar effect in human mothers who consume GMO foods contaminated with the same gene? The mother may do everything in her power such as resting, taking her supplements, looking after herself, but if she is consuming foods that contain a "killer gene," then her unborn child is at risk.

For families struggling to become pregnant, it would be simple to change to an organic diet if it will reduce the risk from contamination via the genetically modified organism.

Issue #4: The discovery of a "new" and toxic gene called 'Gene VI', that now lurks in 54 of 86 GM crops, is being tested. This gene may be responsible for miscarriages of pregnant animals and humans.

Chapter Summary

Genetically modified crops and the foods derived from them are a real threat to human health and wellbeing. The risks to your colon health and digestive health are more important to us in this book precisely because these products are eaten. They enter the body via the mouth and who knows the extent of the damage they cause all throughout the digestive system and intestinal tract until they leave the body?

We looked at four main issues that you need to be mindful of when selecting foods for your consumption and for your loved ones.

I also want you to be able to put a proper system in place, whereby you can enjoy the best of life with assurance that you are doing your part.

Chapter References

[1] http://listverse.com/2008/04/01/top-10-bizarre-genetically-modified-organisms/

[2] http://www.cban.ca/Resources/Topics/GE-Crops-and-Foods-On-the-Market

[3] http://news.cahnrs.wsu.edu/2012/10/01/summary-of-major-findings-and-definitions-of-important-terms/

[4] Genetic Roulette The Movie

[5] Dangers of GM Fish,
http://www.hippocratesinst.org/2012-09/the-dangers-of-gm-fish

[6] http://www.cbc.ca/news/health/story/2010/09/10/pei-gmo-salmon-aquabounty-584.html

[7]http://www.dailymail.co.uk/news/article-2266143/Uncovered-toxic-gene-hiding-GM-crops-Revelation-throws-new-doubt-safety-foods.html?ito=feeds-newsxml

* * * * *

Children and Colon Health

Chapter 10

* * *

"Train up a child in the path when he is young and he will not depart from it when he is old." - Holy Scripture

"A child's health is so fragile and every parent needs to become knowledgeable about digestive and colon health, if only for the sake of their children." - Jenny Berkeley, RN, Certified Holistic Nutritionist

* * *

In my over-two decades in nursing, I have had the chance to see many young patients brought into the hospital emergency room (ER) from as young as a year old. I always spend time speaking to the parents asking questions to try to understand their own level of knowledge or ignorance about basic principles of holistic health.

I've seen children brought in for common colds and parents expecting doctors to fix it with a magic pill or injection. I've also seen children brought in with much more serious conditions.

Whatever the reason for the child coming into the ER, the expression on every parent is always the same. They are filled with fear, worry, concern, and want their child to be better. That is what every parent wants, isn't it?

Parents want their children to be in good health. I think this is especially so for the mother who laboured for nine months carrying the child. She went through all the morning sickness, the terrible food cravings, the mood swings, the highs and the lows, and the post-partum depression. Mothers have a special connection. Fathers still have a bond as well, but it is not the same as a mother's.

So let me start by asking a few questions for you to think about.

Which is better, to treat a sickness once it has started or to not become sick in the first place?

Which is harder, to swallow medication that tastes awful and makes you feel nauseous or to eat food that tastes good and will make you feel contented?

Which is easier, to live each day with pain in your joints or to drink 2 to 3 litres of water a day?

I can tell you that perhaps 99 of 100 people who read those questions will all answer them the way you probably just did.

They will say that not becoming sick in the first place is the better option.

They will say that taking the medication that is awful is the harder option.

They will say that drinking 2 to 3 litres of water a day is the easier option.

They have all answered it correctly from a rational way of thinking. And if your answers were the same, you too answered correctly from a rational way of thinking.

Yet, even if they all know the correct answer, they will fail to follow through with it on an emotional level. There is something which is disconnected between the rational ideal and the implementation.

The Children Make the Difference

While most people will not make the change for themselves, they will make the change for their children. If a family of one boy and two girls finds out that the latest child has an allergy to nuts, then the parents will make the entire family a nut-free family. The other children who are not allergic will not be allowed to bring nuts into the house even if they are allowed to eat them outside.

Now suppose the allergy was dairy, instead of nuts. The same procedure would be followed. The entire family would be dairy-free in the home. For the sake of the health of one child, the entire family would adopt a lifestyle inside the home that is beneficial for the child.

One story that comes to mind is that of Victoria Boutenko. She was a Russian immigrant who came to America with her husband and two young children after the fall of the Berlin Wall. When they first came to America they were amazed by the amount of food in the supermarket. There was such an abundance of food items that they wanted to try everything in the store.

Not long after, Victoria, her husband, and the children, began to come down with various Western illnesses. But the turning point for Victoria was when she learned that her son was a diabetic and would be forced to take insulin shots for the rest of his life. Victoria was deathly scared of the thought of her son taking those insulin shots. She had experienced another relative who was close to her dying due to the diabetic condition.

This experience had left such an indelible imprint on Victoria's mind that the pronouncement of diabetes was to her the same as a death sentence. And Victoria did not want this for her son whom she loved dearly.

With that tipping point Victoria began her search for a means to cure her son from this death sentence called diabetes. She was like a frantic woman. Another story she relates is standing on a street corner and looking at people who seemed healthy and stopping them to ask them if they knew about health and could talk to her.

Some people might have thought she was a crazy woman while others might have simply passed on by. But as fate would have it, she happened to encounter the person who Victoria thought might have been the only raw fooder in the entire state at the time. She asked this lady whether she knew about health and would she be willing to tell her over a cup of coffee. The woman replied that she did know about health and would tell Victoria, but would not drink coffee because she did not eat the same foods that Victoria did.

Victoria listened to the woman and learned from the woman about a living food diet and lifestyle. Victoria's son eventually was declared no longer diabetic. Victoria's other family members also saw benefits to changing their diet and lifestyle. And Victoria went on to write books and promote this lifestyle to others around the globe.

I was introduced to the living foods concept by a friend giving me one of Victoria's books. And so you see, the love of a mother can influence the world.

Infants and Colon Health

I know of a story of a parent who, many years ago, went to visit a paediatrician about her sick child.

The parent had gone to see the paediatrician because of concerns that her infant had not had a bowel movement in three days. The parent was naturally a bit concerned about this, especially since the child was cranky because of it.

The paediatrician simply smiled at the mother and told her not to worry. She said that this is perfectly normal and that she had seen cases where the infant had not had a bowel movement for as long as days. As you can imagine, the parent was in disbelief. If one can imagine how awful it feels as an adult to go three or four days without a bowel movement, then how awful it must be for the infant who is unable to say so. The parent persisted and asked the doctor for anything that could be done. And the doctor recommended something to try if the child had not had any movements in the next 24 hours.

This story can be the story of most parents today. They think it is normal for a one-year-old or 18-month-old to have infrequent bowel movements. Yet I can tell you that infants should have at the very least one to two bowel movements per day. They can have more, which is perfectly normal for an infant.

If it is more than 24 hours and the child has not had a bowel movement, then I would say the child is already showing signs of constipation.

Now it is time for the parent to put on the hat of a private detective and attempt to figure out why the child is not having proper bowel movements. It could be that the child is suffering from allergies to the formula. Or perhaps the child is dehydrated from not enough moisture and water. Or maybe the parents need to massage the infant's tummy each day.

To figure out if it is related to the formula, consult someone who is able to assess whether your child is allergic to dairy or soy. Also, make sure the formula you are using is organic and GMO free.

At the time a child is more than one year old, I would suggest making a routine of giving the child some water to drink each day. This water needs to be boiled and sterilized first. It is a good idea to boil a batch of water and set it aside to cool to room temperature for the child. Then give the child a few ounces just before her regular feedings when she is hungry. She will drink the water and then you can give the bottle. For breast feeding mothers, you can still give the child a bit of water before the breast.

If the child needs the parent to gently rub the tummy, then take a few minutes to rub the tummy gently. Consider it bonding time with the child.

Children and Colon Health

From the time the child is about 3 years old and able to communicate verbally and understand you, it is time to begin teaching the child sound digestive health principles.

The things you must teach the child include:
- When to eat.
- When to drink.
- When to poop.
- How to poop.
- What foods to avoid.
- Which foods are healthy.

I see in some schools the food routine they have set up and I believe that these are indeed set up for the benefit of the food industry and not the benefit of human health.

For example, one big error that I find is that children are being conditioned to eat constantly. And I see this in the elementary school system. Children wake up in the morning and have breakfast by 8 a.m., then they eat a snack at 10, then lunch at 12, then snack at 2, then dinner at 6 p.m. So children would have eaten 4 to 6 times in a day on a typical school day. Is it any wonder our nation's children struggle with weight issues?

The problem with eating all day like that is that it never gives the internal organs connected with the digestive system a time to rest. I see that it will create an internal fatigue in the liver, pancreas, the colon, and overall in the child because the body needs rest time.

As a parent, you need to not follow the rest down the wrong path. Teach your child the right time to eat and let the school know this is your desire for the child.

A child can eat 3 times a day with no snacking in between

meals. A snack is a meal according to the brain and the body. The brain does not place labels like lunch, dinner, snack, on things we eat. The brain only knows food or not, drink or not. Thus a snack is food. A soup is food. A smoothie is food (but liquid food). A coffee with lots of milk and sugar is FOOD in a liquid form like a soup. A drink with lots of sugar and flavour is a liquid food.

So parents can teach the child to eat only three times a day to help them control their appetite.

When to drink

Children should be taught to never drink with their meals. I see children sitting at lunch with their glasses of milk or juice next to their food and I think, "oh my". I see all these children as becoming potential stomach- and digestive-issue patients in their early 20's, 30's, and 40's. This is the natural outcome of habitually hurting the digestive system every day. In other chapters in this book I outline the best method to approach drinking. The same principles apply to children.

When and How to Poop

What people typically call "potty training" is actually what I call "potty untraining." What do I mean by this? Let me illustrate this with a story. Take a perfectly healthy woman and teach her to walk with a limp. Show her this and tell her this is the only way to walk. Now when you see this woman walking along with a limp, this would be weird. If you knew she was perfectly healthy, then why should she limp, correct? It is just insane. But here is the other thing. If she continues to walk with that limp for 20 or 30 years, then she will make her body develop that limp permanently.

Now when parents begin to potty untrain their child, they are essentially teaching a healthy human being to poop with a limp. And it will be something that will stick with the child for the rest of their lives, ensuring that they develop colon issues in their 60's, 70's and 80's. Of course, this is dependent on a variety of diet and lifestyle factors which can expedite or slow the onset of the dis-ease.

Western sitting-style toilets are designed for sick people to poop, not for healthy people. I have arrived at this conclusion after years of consideration of the matter. Squatting toilets like the ones in India or parts of Asia are the toilets designed for healthy individuals.

The proper way to train a child to poop is by the use of the squatting position. This is healthful for the calves, thighs, lower back, and the colon. It makes pooping quick and uneventful. There is no straining or waiting.

Pooping should be trained into a habit of early morning. Always ask the children to try to poop in the morning before going to school. You may need to ask them shortly after waking and again just before leaving the house. This is important because children may be self-conscious and not want to poop in school during the day. Thus by having them poop in the morning, you are giving their body a chance to release the waste and toxins. Have them squat and try to poop even if they say they don't feel like it. You would be amazed just by the act of attempting to poop, that some poop will come out.

Then again have them try to poop before bedtime.

What foods to eat and what to avoid

Children need a wholesome, healthy diet. I would never recommend that candy be given to children, even recreationally. There is really no purpose for candy in the diet of kids. There is no need for lollipops, sweets, chewing gum, chocolate-coated anything like nuts, raisins, or the like.

The basic principle of health and wellness is that good food will help the body to perform better. However, in order to eat good food, they need not be processed to death.

Give your children more fresh fruits, vegetables, greens, smoothies, and some nuts and seeds. There are literally hundreds of things you can make with these items and a good high-speed blender.

Foods that should be avoided include dairy, meats, processed sweets and candies, and sugary drinks. When you introduce these foods to your children too soon, they become hooked on the taste of them. Parents must guide children into what is helpful for health and strength and what is not.

They need to think of it like training a child who has allergies to certain foods. From a very early age, a parent teaches the child what foods to avoid because they are allergic. The parent knows that the child's health depends on recognizing the bad foods and not accepting them from friends or eating them accidentally.

Parents can teach children from as young as four to read a produce bar code and look for the number "9" for organic, "8" for GMOs, and "3" for conventionally grown produce.

Avoid all GMOs. Avoid conventionally grown foods as much as possible. Do not introduce these toxic-laden foods to your children if you can avoid it.

Teens and Colon Health

For teens, you need to give them a more detailed explanation of why they need to avoid foods which make them sick. The challenge is that some teens do not want to listen to their parents because they are at an age where they believe they know better.

If a parent can convince their teenager to do voluntary work in a hospital for a couple of months, then it will make a huge difference in their understanding of the nature of disease. It takes a concept that is not real, the concept of sickness, to them and makes it very real.

Teens need foods that build their mind and strengthen their capacity for intellectual thinking. But, they also need to eat foods that clean and clear out their colon because toxins that remain in the colon find their way back into the bloodstream and impact the brain.

A clean colon also helps with healthier skin. Parents of teenage girls dealing with acne and skin blemishes can help them by encouraging them to eat a high raw diet loaded with colon-cleansing fibre.

My most heartbreaking experiences are when I see a teenager between 15 and 19 with severe colon issues or even condemned to a colostomy bag. That is a bag connected to your colon so that poop comes out the side of your stomach via a tube into the plastic bag. It needs to be changed regularly and it can smell. A procedure like this for a teenager will impact their self-esteem all through their adult years. It will make them feel self conscious, inadequate, ugly, or unworthy of love. This is on top of all the other things young people have to deal with in their lives.

So I encourage parents to get educated on the topic and have candid discussions with their teens about their colon, their stomach, and anything that hurts, feels uncomfortable, or is not right.

Chapter Summary

In this chapter we looked at the importance of colon health from birth right up into the teenage years. I highlighted for you some of the key functions I believe are necessary for any parent to teach their children in order to maintain a healthy, functioning colon well into their adult years.

* * * * *

Comfort Food and Discomforting Trap

Chapter 11

* * *

"In one imagines the brain as a personal computer and the eyes as a kind of solar panel that charges and stores its energy source, one becomes aware of an intuition that all life forms contain. Therefore, living "sun-cooked" food is like minisolar batteries that fuel the human physical machine with life force essence." - Rev. Viktoras Kulvinskas, MS

"Comfort Food is a contradiction. Food is for strength and vitality. When people look to food for comfort, they will ultimately become a slave to that food like a drug addict is a slave to the drug." - Jenny Berkeley, RN, Certified Holistic Nutritionist

* * *

For almost every human being in the world, there is some food that gives them a sense of comfort. This food from their adult years or childhood often brings to mind some emotions of calm or joy and so they eat these foods when they feel they need a pickup or boost.

One large fast food restaurant has actually been trying for decades to make its food become a comfort food for kids and adults. This is so that those people will always run back to buy the restaurant's food whenever they feel they need an emotional boost. Do you know of the "happy meal"? By naming it a happy meal and having parents give it to their children, it is trying to create that emotional (irrational) bond between being happy and eating that unhealthy meal.

Here is another example: an adult male with mood swings who when he has a really bad day or week, will turn to white bread, cheese, meats, and eat them. He says he knows these are not good for him but he was so stressed out.

But my teaching is happiness is your good health, and your health is your wealth. So in this chapter we'll look at ways to try and break the emotional food-eating cycle.

Ways to Comfort Yourself Without Comfort Foods

Using Spiritual / Divine Connections

The world has a few billion people of different religious beliefs. A source of comfort overlooked with many religious believers is a relationship to their god. I write in this section from a Judeo/Christian perspective but the principle is applicable to any spiritual beliefs.

Prayer: Prayer is the way that believers communicate with the God of heaven and earth. Prayer is telling God, Hashem, Yahweh, or Jesus, the things on your mind that bother you and concern you. And it is quietly listening for him to give you an answer to your prayer and concern. Training yourself to be prayerful instead of reaching for that donut, chocolate, or unhealthy food is much better in the long run.

Bible Verse Meditation: The holy scriptures are filled with verses that help to quiet the mind and comfort the soul. For example, "yea though I walk through the valley of death, I shall fear no evil, because you are with me," or "love your god with all your heart, this is the first great command, and the second is like it, love your neighbour as you love yourself." If you write 5 new bible verses each week on an index card and keep them in your wallet, then pull them out and read them when you feel stressed, you will have a meditation that can help calm your mind. I say 5 new ones each week because people tend to get lazy if things get familiar. By picking 5 new verses each week, it is always new and fresh and useful when you feel stressed.

Silent Meditation: A silent meditation is one of the most beneficial things a person can do. While you think on the God of heaven and earth in the silence around you, you will begin to quiet your mind. Unfortunately in today's "always on" world, it is difficult to find that time alone. And this time is necessary long before you have a stressful situation. Try in the early hours of the morning, like 4 a.m.

Talking With Your Spiritual Partner: Most people don't recognize that they have a spiritual partner on their journey. While children are growing up, their spiritual partners are their parents, or uncles, or aunts, who are helping them understand more about their relationship to God. As adults, it may be a spouse, partner, boyfriend, or girlfriend who takes on that role.

Using Mental Exercises and Training

Aside from the spiritual methods to calm yourself so that you are not tempted to use food as a comfort mechanism, you can also do mental exercises to strengthen your mind.

Affirmations: Affirmations are statements that you repeat to yourself or in the presence of others to help you position yourself mentally for the day or the challenge ahead of you. Affirmations are very effective and you might have seen them in the movies without even realizing you were seeing affirmations. Some examples include, "Go Joe (GI Joe Movie)", "I Live For This" (Triple X), "Yippie Kai Yay" (Die Hard Movie), and so on. These short lines signalled that the person saying it was ready for action. And saying it before taking action was the affirmation. But there are also affirmations used in everyday situations like the student who tells herself, "I'm so ready for this exam" or the student who says "I am ready to win this game." Even professional sporting athletes use affirmations before a game to motivate themselves. If the military, movies, and students use affirmations, then there is something valuable to their use. Use them instead of food.

Optimism: Optimism is believing that the world is a better place. When some people eat chocolate they might believe the world is a better place, but that is only until the biochemical reaction of the chocolate wears out. A better and more permanent way to keep that view is by purposely being optimistic. By looking for good in the world, in people you know, and in yourself, you can position your mind to be optimistic about life.

Daydreaming: Daydreaming is one other way to help you avoid those comfort foods. Sometimes it helps to use your imagination to help you picture those things you'd like. How about thinking of yourself on a nice, warm, sunny beach in the middle of a hectic workday in winter? Just spending a few moments there in your mind can help you feel a lot better. Or perhaps reliving a memory of your last beach visit and making it even better. You could use a car you like, a place you'd like to visit, or anything else to help you daydream. Don't do this too often as it becomes a form of escapism if it prevents you from getting productive work done.

Read a Familiar Book: A book is an extremely awesome way to boost your mood. If the book has happy stories or stories of remarkable human beings, then it can help you be optimistic. As it has a fixed beginning and end, it can help you daydream about the story but at the same time put a time limit on it so you don't waste too much time. Developing a habit of reading a good book is essential for you.

Physical Comfort Connections

Your Teddy or Blanky: The teddy bear or blanky (child's blanket) is a symbol of the comfort article that a child uses to help them feel better about their life. Even adults have such a thing. There are the lucky rabbit's foot (which is not so lucky for the rabbit), the lucky coin (which has no value unless it is spent), the lucky horseshoe, or lucky underwear, any other item that a person can hold on to when stressed. I would say that these should only be short-term items because they can be lost, stolen, or taken away. But they can be helpful in the short term and as children grow out of their blanky, so adults grow out of their lucky whatever. Short-term use only.

Exercise: Exercise is one of the better physical comfort tools you can use. It has numerous beneficial impacts on the body, both physically and mentally. Exercise like walking helps a person to focus on other things instead of their own worries. Exercise has also been shown to reduce stress, depression, and feelings of being sluggish. Exercise also boosts the "happy hormones" produced by the body. It brings more oxygen into the body and helps to move toxins around and out of the body. A nice, brisk walk will also help with bowel movements as the impact of gravity and your feet pounding the floor helps the stool to move.

Warm Bath: This is another excellent way to comfort yourself instead of reaching for comfort foods. A nice, warm bath where you just relax and soak almost feels like your troubles are soaking away. It is great when you have the time and need to de-stress. If you use some of your favourite scented oils, you can make the experience even better. When you are in a bath, you won't be thinking of any comfort foods.

Aroma Therapy: This is another way to help soothe your mind. Using your sense of smell to fill your mind with pleasant aromas is great. I would not recommend any synthetic chemicals. Use fresh flowers, or the smell of fresh fruit, or even oils made from plants.

Massage: This is another great way to relax your mind and body. It can be expensive to go to a professional masseuse, so if that is not in your budget, you could have a family member, spouse, or close friend help you out with a massage. It does not have to be a full body massage. Simply massaging the hands and feet can bring tremendous benefit to the person.

<u>The Direct Approach</u>

We have spent the earlier part of this chapter discussing ways to deal with the stress and anguish so that you do not need to rush out for that piece of comfort food. In this section, we look at eliminating the source of the stress because if you keep going back to the stress source, then you will always feel like you need to be comforted with your comfort item (food in this case).

Confront The Source of Your Discomfort: The source of your distress could be your job on a larger level, or your boss, on a smaller level, or your co-worker on a micro level. Think of the entire situation. If your problem is your co-worker, try being nice to them or have a third party mediate the conflict. If the problem is your boss, then have a discussion about it, then with a mediator. If mediation fails, then perhaps it is time to consider a change of jobs. It could be a sign that you're not really meant for that job at this time in your life. If fear of being unemployed is the only thing keeping you at your job, then you really don't have a reason to stay there. It will make you sick. A person should be glad to be at their job. It should add joy and enrichment to the person. Otherwise it is adding pain.

Join A Support Group and Talk About It: Sometimes the job is not the problem. It could be an unhealthy learned habit like gambling, alcoholism, drugs, binge eating/drinking, or some other source of your distress. These things may be the source of your distress, the result of your distress, or both. Like a vicious cycle that keeps repeating itself over and over. The only way to break the cycle is to bring in an external entity experienced in dealing with the situation. Try a support group that is capable of helping you cope with and overcome those issues.

Work Through The Issue With a Counsellor: Sometimes the issues you are dealing with may not be suitable for a group setting. But they are still causing you distress and causing you to go towards eating your comfort foods. This is when you need to see a person one-to-one with experience in helping others in such circumstances. Perhaps a priest, pastor, or counsellor can help you in that situation.

Chapter Summary

In this chapter we talked a bit about the comfort foods and some of the reasons people gravitate towards them. Most importantly, I provided you with a few ideas to help you avoid having to turn to unhealthy comfort foods for emotional support.

* * * * *

Plant-based Recipes

Chapter 12

* * *

"In one imagines the brain as a personal computer and the eyes as a kind of solar panel that charges and stores its energy source, one becomes aware of an intuition that all life forms contain. Therefore, living "sun-cooked" food is like minisolar batteries that fuel the human physical machine with life force essence." - Rev. Viktoras Kulvinskas, MS

"Comfort Food is a contradiction. Food is for strength and vitality. When people look to food for comfort, they will ultimately become a slave to that food like a drug addict is a slave to the drug." - Jenny Berkeley, RN, Certified Holistic Nutritionist

* * *

Featured Recipes

BREAKFAST
- Quinoa Kheer
- Hemp Quinoa Cereal
- Maple Coconut Granola

DRINKS
- Gingery Barley Pears
- Goji Hemp Bliss Milkshake
- Vanilla Sweet Almond

SOUPS
- Spicy Lentil & Kale Soup
- Indo-Canadian Dahl Soup

LUNCH/DINNER
- Sweet Potato Humus Wrap
- Millet Mash-Up
- Beet Pesto Pasta
- Black-eyed Pea Stew With Tempeh
- Almond Coconut Pasta

SALADS
- Chermoula Chickpea Salad
- Coleslaw Chickpea Mix
- Raw Goodness Probiotic Slaw
- Raw Tabbouleh

In addition to the recipes, bear in mind that a healthful lifestyle for your colon by design would involve freshly made fruit and vegetable juices daily.

A NOTE ON DESSERTS:
Jenny has a collection of some of her most delicious desserts in her book Sweet RAW Desserts: Life Is Sweet Raw! They are raw foods desserts that are delicious. Get the book and try them yourself.

Quinoa Kheer

What is Kheer? in Hindi it denotes sweet Indian rice pudding made by boiling rice, milk, sugar, flavoured with cardamom, saffron, almonds, cashews, pistachio and raisins. It is usually served as a dessert and it is very popular during the festival seasons. You can eat it as a dessert or a breakfast meal.

For our version, we're making it vegan and adding other spices to give it a delicious taste.

Ingredients
1   cup   quinoa grains
½   cup   coconut milk
½   cup   water
1½ cup   almond milk
1   pinch saffron
1   tsp   cinnamon powder
¼   tsp   nutmeg powder
2   pods cardamom
½   cup   raw almonds chopped
½   cup   raw pistachio chopped
2   tbsp sprouted chia and flax powder
4   tbsp coconut sugar or yacon syrup
¼   cup   figs, diced into cube
2   cup   almond milk
1   pinch sea salt

Procedure
1. Sprout (for raw version) or Cook Quinoa (non-raw)
2. Sprout -- to make 2 cups of sprouted quinoa, put 1 ½ cup of quinoa in a mason jar filled with cool filtered water.
3. Soak for 30 minutes, then drain off the water.
4. Rinse quinoa well several times.
5. Place a mesh lids on the jar and set it over the counter top at room temperature.
6. Rinse and drain again every 12 hours until tail are formed.
7. Now it is ready to use.

8. Cook--- Rinse the sprouted quinoa first several time. Combine water, coconut milk, almond milk, cardamom pods, saffron and quinoa in a medium sized pot. Bring to a boil over medium heat than reduce to low heat and simmer for 15 minutes or until most of the liquid is absorbed. Turn off the heat and let it cool down.
9. After cooking the quinoa, add the coconut sugar, cinnamon powder, nutmeg powder, almonds, pistachios,figs, sea salt, and sprouted chia and flax meal together.
10. Then add almond milk a little at a time until all the liquid is absorbed and you will have a pudding consistency.
11. You can add more almond milk and top with additional nuts and figs.

Servings: 4
Yield: 4

Degree of Difficulty: Very easy

Preparation Time: 15 minutes
Inactive Time: 12 hours

Cooking Time: 15 minutes
Total Time: 12 hours and 30 minutes

Hemp Quinoa Cereal

Hemp foods have been popular these days and seems to be popping out of every cereal box. Hemp seeds are mighty tiny foods and nutritional powerhouses delivering complete nutrients profile; loaded with protein, essential fatty acids, antioxidants, chlorophyll and other vitamins and minerals.. They are loaded with complete protein, a mere 2 tablespoons dishing up to 11 grams of protein! While Quinoa is also an excellent protein and is high in calcium, iron, and phosphorous.

Ingredients

1	cup	red quinoa
2	cups	hemp milk
½	tsp	vanilla powder
1	tsp	cinnamon powder
¼	cup	coconut sugar or coconut nectar
1	pinch	sea salt
1	cup	mixed berries
1		bananas, sliced
2	tbsp	hemp nuts
1/4	cup	pecans chopped or almonds sliced

Procedure
1. Sprout the red quinoa in cool water for 6 hours until small tail are seen. Rinse off the quinoa several times and drain in the colander.
2. Combine the sprouted quinoa with hemp milk, cinnamon powder, vanilla powder, coconut sugar and sea salt in a medium pot over medium heat.
3. Let it cook while stirring often until simmered.
4. Cover, reduce heat to low and cook the quinoa for 20 minutes until the liquid is absorbed.
5. Let the quinoa cereal cool down for 5 minutes than add fresh berries, banana sliced, hemp nuts and chopped pecans.
6. Serve warm.

Servings: 4
Yield: 4

Degree of Difficulty: Very easy
Preparation Time: 20 minutes

Cooking Time: 20 minutes
Inactive Time: 6 hours

Total Time: 6 hours and 20 minutes

Maple Coconut Granola

Granola are easy to make and a great handy snack to have around in your pantry cupboard. It is great for breakfast, you can create as colourful as you want by adding fruit sauce, coconut whipped cream, fresh fruits, or vegan yogurt.

Ingredients

2	cups	gluten free rolled oat
1/4	cup	almonds, finely diced
1/4	cup	sunflower seeds
1/4	cup	pumpkin seeds
1/4	cup	raisins
1/4	cup	cranberries
1/8	cup	Goji berries
1	tbsp	cinnamon powder
1/4	tsp	nutmeg powder
1/4	tsp	clove powder
1	tsp	vanilla powder
1/4	tsp	sea salt
1/4	cup	water
1/4	cup	dates, pitted
1/4	cup	coconut milk
2	tbsp	coconut oil
1/2	cup	Maple syrup

Procedure
1. Soak the dates in the 1/4 cup of water until soft.
2. In a large bowl combine rolled oats, almonds, sunflower seeds, pumpkin seeds, raisins, cranberries, goji berries, salt, vanilla powder, cinnamon powder, nutmeg and clove powder.
3. Transfer the soaked dates with water to the blender.
4. Blend until smooth, then add coconut milk, maple syrup and coconut oil. Blend again until it is smooth.
5. Pour the mixture onto the dry ingredients and thoroughly mixed them well.
6. Preheat the oven to 350F.

7. Transfer the granola to lined baking pan and bake for 40 minutes while turning evenly every 10 minutes to make sure is evenly golden brown.
8. Let stand for 5 to 10 minutes to allow to cool down.
9. Transfer to air tight container.

Servings: 6
Yield: 6

Degree of Difficulty: Very easy
Preparation Time: 10 minutes

Cooking Time: 40 minutes
Total Time: 50 minutes

Gingery Barley Pears

Barley grass provide the life force of health benefit. It is high in antioxidants, vitamins A, E, folate, protein, minerals including potassium, iron, magnesium, calcium, manganese, essential amino acids, chlorophyll and high level of enzymatic activity that is necessary for building new, strong, healthy and vital cells in the body.

Moringa is one of the most nutrient rich plants on planet earth. Very high in protein, Vitamin A, Calcium, potassium,magnesium, iron, zinc and contains all the essential amino acids. It is one of my best superfoods.

Ingredients
2   ripe pear
2   frozen bananas
1   tsp   grated ginger
2   cups water or coconut water
2   cups baby spinach
1   tsp   moringa powder
1   tsp   barley powder
1   tsp   lemon juice

Procedure
10. Blend all ingredients together until smooth and creamy.
11. Taste and adjust sweetness as desired.

Servings: 2
Yield: 16 oz

Degree of Difficulty: Very easy
Preparation Time: 10 minutes

Total Time: 10 minutes

Goji Hemp Bliss Milkshake

Goji berries are another nutritional powerhouse. They are rich in protein with eighteen amino acids, including the eight essential amino acids that make up a complete protein. They are very high in antioxdiants, rich in Vitamin A and vitamin C. They are better sources of vitamin C than oranges. You can boost your immunity by just adding goji berries in your diet.

Add it to cold or hot cereal, smoothies, desserts, baked goods, sprinkle on salads, cooked in soup. As a child, I remember my mom would always cook this tonic soup filled with goji berries and it tasted so delicious. Now I appreciate the value of adding this superfood powerhouse to my diet.

Ingredients
2   cups almond mylk
¼   cup Goji berries
½   cup hemp nuts
1   tsp   cinnamon powder
4   dates, pitted

Procedure
1. Soak goji berries and dates in almonds mylk for 30 minutes.
2. Transfer to the blender with the rest of the ingredients and blend for 15 seconds until is smooth and creamy.
3. Pour into two tall glass and serve chilled.

Servings: 2
Yield: 2

Degree of Difficulty: Very easy
Preparation Time: 15 minutes

Total Time: 15 minutes

Vanilla Sweet Almond Mylkshake

This milkshake just melts in your mouth, so silky and creamy! Some of the raw protein powders have a grainy texture but with Sunwarrior vegan powder, there is no grainy texture! I remember the first time I drank this milkshake. It was so smooth, silky and creamy. The feeling made me remember the traditional milkshake filled with heavy cream but this version is free from the fear of clogged arteries.

Ingredients
2   cups   almond milk
2   frozen bananas
½ tsp   vanilla powder
½ tsp   cinnamon powder
1   tbsp   lucuma powder
1   tbsp   hemp nuts
1   scoop Sunwarrior vanilla raw vegan powder
4   medjool dates, pitted

Procedure
1. Blend all ingredients until smooth and creamy.
2. Taste and adjust sweetener as desired.

Servings: 2
Yield: 16 ounce

Degree of Difficulty: Very easy

Spicy Lentil & Kale Soup

Spicy lentil and Kale soup is a favourite in my house. We'll
usually have it twice in a week when we're in the mood. It is
delicious, quick and a pleaser. If you don't have time to make
vegetable broth than you can use organic vegetable bouillon
cubes, ½ a cube with 6 cups of water.

Ingredients
1	cup	red lentils
2	cups	water
4	tbsp	olive oil
¼	cup	onion coarsely chopped
6		garlic clove, chopped
1	cup	kabocha squash, cubed
¼	cup	celery, chopped
2	large	tomatoes chopped
2		bay leaves
1	tbsp	nama shoyu
1	tsp	coriander powder
1	tsp	cumin powder
1	tsp	paprika powder
1/8	tsp	chipotle pepper
1/8	tsp	cayenne pepper
1	cup	kale leaves chopped
1	pinch	sea salt and black pepper to taste
6	cups	vegetable broth

Procedure
1. Soak red lentils in 2 cups of water for 2 hours.
2. Rinse off the lentils a few times in cool running water
   and drain off excess water.
3. In a large pot combine olive oil, garlic, onion, bay leaf,
   cumin, coriander, paprika, cayenne pepper, chipotle
   pepper, kabocha squash, tomatoes and nama shoyu to
   sauté for 10 minutes, then add the lentils with 6 cups of
   vegetable broth and simmer for 20 minutes until the
   lentils are cooked.
4. Stir in kale leaves to cook for another 5 minutes.
5. Season with salt and black pepper to taste.

Servings: 4
Yield: 4
Degree of Difficulty: Very easy
Preparation Time: 15 minutes

Cooking Time: 30 minutes
Total Time: 45 minutes

Indo-Canadian Dahl Soup

Dahl is one of my favourite soups. It is such a satisfying hearty soup especially during the cold winter months. I remember in my native country, this soup was made so watery and spicy. I adapted a Canadian version and added more seasonings to bring out the richness of flavours.

Ingredients
2 cups yellow split peas
8 cups water
¼ cup onion coarsely chopped
3 garlic clove, chopped
1 tsp cumin powder
1 tsp coriander powder
3 tbsp olive oil or coconut oil
2 tomato chopped
½ tsp tumeric powder
1 tsp sea salt
½ cup cilantro chopped

Procedure
1. Presoak the yellow split peas overnight for 12 hours to cut down the cooking time and also sprouting the peas will help with digestion process.
2. Rinse off the peas in a cool running water.
3. Place the peas and water in a large pot over high heat for 30 minutes then lower to medium heat for 1 hour and 15 minutes.
4. Cook the split peas until soft or tender. Stir regularly to check consistency is creamy. Turn off and allow to cool.

5. In a large skillet, combine olive oil, garlic, onion, cilantro, tomato, sea salt, cumin powder and coriander powder. Saute for 10 minutes. Allow to cool to room temperature.
6. Pour this sauteed seasoning over cooked split peas soup and stir the soup.
7. Garnish with chopped cilantro. Serve with brown rice.

Servings: 8
Yield: 8
Degree of Difficulty: Very easy
Preparation Time: 15 minutes
Cooking Time: 2 hours
Inactive Time: 12 hours

Sweet Potato Humus Wrap

Collard greens has a milder flavour than any other winter greens. It make such a wonderful alternative to flour-based wraps. It is packed with foliate, B vitamin that may help lessen the risk of hypertension. Sweet potatoes orange hue is the beautiful result of bountiful of beta-carotene, which helps support eye health and boost the immunity. Serve this as a dip with crisp-tender vegetables such as red peppers, celery, broccoli, cucumber and carrots. You will get an extra boost of Vitamin C, selenium and sulforaphane.

Ingredients
4	med	sweet potato, peeled and cubed
1 ½	cup	cooked chickpeas
¼	cup	tahini butter
¼	cup	extra virgin olive oil
½		lemon juice
½	tsp	paprika powder
½	tsp	cumin powder
¼	tsp	sea salt
¼	tsp	black pepper freshly ground
1		avocado, thinly sliced
8	large	collard leaves
1	cup	red pepper, cut into strips
1		carrot, slice into matchsticks
2	cups	microgreen sprouts

Procedure
1. Place sweet potatoes in streamer basket and stream until very tender for 20 minutes. Set aside to cool.
2. Place cooked sweet potatoes and chickpeas in food processor and blend together.
3. Add tahini, garlic, olive oil, lemon juice, paprika, cumin, sea salt and black pepper. Blend until smooth.
4. To prepare the wraps: cut off the white stalks of the collards. Fillet off the thickest parts of stalks that run down the leave with a sharp knife , try not to nick off the leaf as you do this.

5. Place 2 collard leaves and add a generous amount of sweet potato humus down the centre lengthwise and then top with avocado, sweet pepper, carrot sticks and microgreens.
6. Tightly roll leaves beginning from the bottom, tucking inside as you go.
7. Cut into half to serve.

Servings: 4
Yield: 4

Degree of Difficulty: Very easy
Preparation Time: 20 minutes

Cooking Time: 20 minutes
Total Time: 40 minutes

Millet Mash-Up

Millet is a nutritionally rich tiny grain which is gluten free and has been a staple food in Asia and India for 10,000 years. They come in different sizes and colours (white, yellow, red and gray). It can be used instead of brown rice or white rice.

Ingredients
1   cup   millet grains
3   cups   vegetable broth
3   cups   cauliflower florets
2   tbsp   extra-virgin olive oil
1   garlic clove, chopped
1   small onion coarsely chopped
1   tsp   sea salt
2   tbsp   chives chopped
½   tsp   black pepper freshly ground

Procedure
1. In a large skillet add olive oil, onion and garlic. Saute over medium heat until the onions are translucent for about 3 minutes.

2. Add the millet, vegetable broth, cauliflowers and salt.
   Bring to a boil over high heat then reduce to low heat
   cover and simmer for 35-40 minutes, until all the
   vegetables are soft and the millet is cooked.
3. Remove from heat and let it cool down for 15 minutes.
4. Transfer to a food processor and blend until smooth
   and creamy.
5. Serve with your favourite dish or eat it alone as a main
   dish and sprinkle chives and black pepper. You can stir
   in vegan butter for a creamy texture.

Servings: 4
Yield: 4

Degree of Difficulty: Very easy
Preparation Time: 15 minutes

Cooking Time: 45 minutes
Total Time: 1 hour

Beet Pesto Pasta

Here is such a beautiful dish with a "wow" factor, as the
pasta gets a striking vibrant red hue from the beet pesto.
Beets not only come in red but also comes in a range of
colours that can add visual flair and flavour to your culinary
creations. The deep crimson that temporarily stains your
hands or utensils comes with such an abundance of
phytonutrients called betalains. This help fight against free
radical and betalains appear to help in the battle of cancer.

Ingredients
4		red beets, medium
½	cup	walnut halves
½	cup	vegan diaya cheese
2		garlic clove, chopped
½		lemon juice
¼	tsp	red chilles flakes
¼	cup	extra virgin olive oil

¼ tsp   sea salt
½ tsp   black pepper
450 g   whole grain fettuccini or linguini or gluten free
pasta
½ cup   baby spinach

Procedure
1. Place beets in a streamer basket until tender, about 40
    minutes. Set aside to cool down and then rub off the
    skins.
2. Combine garlic, lemon juice, beets, chili flakes, sea salt
    and vegan daiya cheese in a food processor.
3. Blend until beets are pulverized. With the machine
    running, pour the olive oil through the feed tube and
    blend into grainy thick texture.
4. Prepare the pasta according to package instruction.
5. Drain the pasta in a cool running water and then return
    to the pot.
6. Add the beet pesto and make sure the pasta is well
    coated with pesto.
7. Serve pasta garnished with spinach and black pepper.

Servings: 6
Yield: 6

Degree of Difficulty: Very easy
Preparation Time: 20 minutes

Cooking Time: 40 minutes
Total Time: 1 hour

Black-eyed Pea Stew With Tempeh

Pronounced "tem-pay" this traditional food that comes from
Indonesia. It is made from whole soyabeans that is
fermented so it is easy to digest. Now you can find many
variety of tempeh products in health food stores: tempeh
made with only soya beans, tempeh with wild rice, barley,
rice, millet, smoked tempeh, grains tempeh, tempeh bacon,
herbs tempeh, and marinated tempeh in various flavours.

Ingredients

4	cups	cooked black eyed peas
8	oz	tempeh, cut into 1 inch cube
2	tbsp	olive oil
1	tbsp	sesame oil
½	cup	onion chopped
2		garlic clove, chopped
1	cup	carrots, diced
½	cup	green pepper, diced
½	cup	red pepper, diced
½	cup	yellow pepper,diced
2		tomatoes, chopped
1	tbsp	cumin powder
1	tbsp	dried oregano
1	tsp	allspice
1	tsp	sea salt
1	tsp	chipotle pepper powder
2	tsp	homemade vegan broth powder

Procedure
1. In a large pot over the medium heat, add olive oil, onion, garlic, allspice, cumin, oregano, and sea salt.
2. Saute for 2 minutes, stirring often until the onion and garlic softens.
3. Add carrots, peppers tomatoes, smoked tempeh, cooked black eyed peas and homemade vegan broth powder with 2 cups of water to simmer over low heat for 15 minutes, until it has a stew-like consistency.
4. Add salt and black pepper and more water if it's too dry.
5. Serve plain or top with chopped red onion, cilantro and shredded non-dairy cheese.

Servings: 8
Yield: 8

Degree of Difficulty: Very easy

Preparation Time: 15 minutes
Cooking Time: 45 minutes

Inactive Time: 1 hour
Total Time: 2 hours

Almond Coconutty Pasta

This is such a delicious creamy pasta without any dairy or heavy cream. I just loved coconut version pasta which is vegan and plant based. Note: you can substitute raw coconut milk with 1 can light coconut milk if you cannot make your own.

Ingredients

1	450 g	brown rice pasta
1	cup	broccoli florets, cut into small pieces
2	cups	raw coconut milk
1/3 cup		raw almond butter
2	tbsp	coconut aminos
2	tsp	grated ginger
2		garlic clove, minced
½	tsp	dried red chili flakes
½	cup	cilantro chopped
½	cup	basil leaves
2	tbsp	cilantro chopped
2	tbsp	sliced almonds

Procedure
1. In a large pot, boil pasta until al dente for about 8 minutes.
2. Drain in cool running water and set aside in a bowl.
3. Cut the broccoli florets into small pieces. Meanwhile prepare the sauce, place almond butter, coconut milk, ginger, garlic, basil, red chili flakes, cilantro and nama shoyu.
4. Pour the sauce over the broccoli florets and let it marinate for 10 minutes.
5. Add the broccoli into the pasta and thoroughly coat the pasta.
6. Garnish with cilantro and slice almonds. Spoon into bowls and serve.

Servings: 6
Yield: 6

Degree of Difficulty: Very easy
Preparation Time: 15 minutes

Cooking Time: 10 minutes
Total Time: 25 minutes

Chermoula Chickpea Salad

Chermoula is typically used as a marinade in North African home. There are many ways to prepare chermoula, some use only cilantro, while others include parsley with preserved lemon or just fresh lemon juice. This sauce is great on pasta dishes, bean dishes and added to fresh bowl of garden salad.

Ingredients

1	bunch	fresh cilantro
3		garlic clove, chopped
2	tsp	paprika
½	tsp	coriander powder
1	tsp	cumin powder
1	tsp	grated ginger
¼	tsp	red chili flakes
¼	tsp	sea salt
½		lemon juice, freshly squeezed
3	tbs	olive oil
1		pinch saffron
2	cups	cooked chickpeas
¼	cup	red onion, diced
1	cup	sweet red pepper, diced
½	cup	fresh cilantro chopped
½	cup	fresh parsley, chopped

Procedure
1. In a small bowl combine cooked chickpeas, sweet red pepper, red onion, cilantro and parsley. Set aside.
2. Combine the rest of the ingredients in a food processor, and process to a thick sauce.
3. Pour the chermoula sauce into the prepared chickpeas bowl.
4. Thoroughly mixed well and let sit for 5 minutes. Serve.

Degree of Difficulty: Very easy
Preparation Time: 15 minutes

Cooking Time: 0 minutes
Total Time: 15 minutes

Coleslaw Chickpea Mix

A quick and easy recipe to enjoy when you are in a crunch.

Ingredients
1 cup cooked chickpeas
1 cup purple cabbage, grated
1 cup carrot, grated
1 cup green cabbage, grated
1 tbsp Dijon mustard
1 tbsp nama shoyu
1 tbsp lemon juice, freshly squeezed
½ tsp raw apple cider vinegar
1 Salt and freshly ground black pepper to taste

Procedure
1. In a small bowl, combine all the ingredients.
2. Toss everything and serve.

Degree of Difficulty: Very easy
Preparation Time: 10 minutes

Total Time: 10 minutes

Raw Goodness Probiotic Slaw

Boost your immunity with this probiotic stew. Good for bowel health too.

Ingredients
1 orange beet, grated
1 red beet, grated
1 carrot, grated
2 garlic clove, minced
2 tbps pumpkin seed oil
2 tbsp hemp oil
¼ cup unpasteurized sauerkraut
¼ cup hemp nuts
1 cup kale, chiffonale
1 tbsp sauerkraut liquid

1/8 tsp sea salt

Procedure
1. Washed the beets and peeled off the skin.
2. Combine grated beets, carrots, minced garlic, kale, sauerkraut, sauerkraut liquid, Styriam Gold Pumpkin Seed oil, hemp oil, and sea salt.
3. Mixed the salad thoroughly then sprinkle hemp nuts.

Servings: 4
Yield: 4

Degree of Difficulty: Very easy
Preparation Time: 15 minutes

Total Time: 15 minutes

Raw Tabbouleh

This is a twist to the traditional tabbouleh, with a lighter crisp version. It is quick and easy to prepare.

Ingredients
1   cup cherry tomato, cut into halve
½   medium cauliflower florets, shredded
¼   cup red onion, diced
½   cup fresh parsley, chopped
2   tbsp fresh mint leaves, chopped
3   tbsp lemon juice
1   tsp sea salt
¼   tsp black pepper freshly ground
2   tbps raw olive oil
1   garlic clove, chopped

Procedure
1. Place the cauliflower florets in a food processor.
2. Pulse a few time until it breakdown to tiny chunks.
3. Combine all the ingredients and toss well.
4. Keeps 5 days in the fridge in the fridge in an airtight container.

Preparation Time: 15 minutes

About The Author

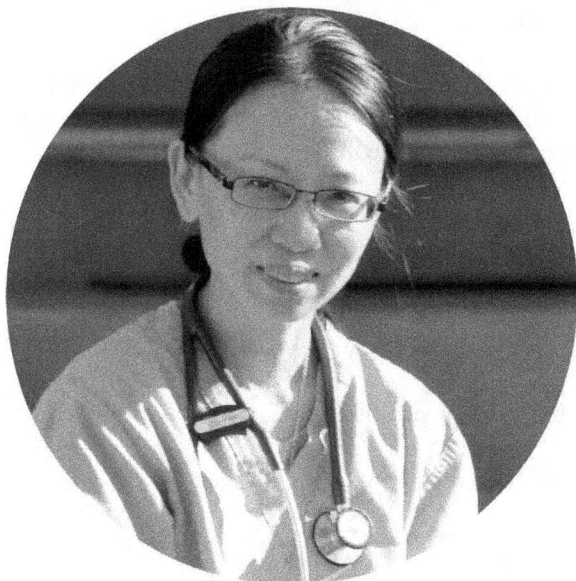

Jenny Berkeley is a registered nurse, a certified holistic nutritionist, a health educator, raw food chef, and best selling kindle author. Jenny is one of Toronto's most connected individuals in the living foods movement. She has worked both locally in Canada and internationally. She is a tiny gal with a big heart that she wears on her sleeve. Jenny has over 22 years of experience in the medical profession caring for her patients, being their advocate, and supporting her colleagues.

In addition to her busy schedule as a medical professional, Jenny still finds the time to do television interviews, radio interviews, and even speak to heads of government on behalf of the organic and living food movement. She goes boldly for the benefit of all Canadian, young and old. She is an author, speaker, lecturer, and blogger. Her Twitter following is almost 40,000. She is also the co-founder and publisher of EternityWatch Magazine, Canada's magazine dedicated to the vegan and raw-vegan community. Her magazine is focused on holistic lifestyle and every issue promotes a holistic approach to health by looking at diet, lifestyle, and your environment. Every issue includes a plant-based recipe for the readers to enjoy.

Her website, Eating4Eternity.org is a wonderful resource for the health-minded that covers topics ranging from square-foot gardening to the living foods.

Facebook: jen.berkeley | Twitter: sproutqueen
Email: info@eating4eternity.org

Amazon Author Page:
http://www.amazon.com/Jenny-Berkeley/e/B00761ML3A

Look for more great titles from The Holistic Health Nurse Series™
www.eating4eternity.org/hhns/

* * * * *

More from CM Berkeley Media Group

CM Berkeley Media Group, based in Canada, works with its authors to produce books which help to uplift the human spirit, spread the message of health and wellness, and offer practical insights in finances, and other areas. We also offer services to help authors convert their books to Kindle or ePUB format, get their book edited, and get a great cover design, and other services for independent authors.

Facebook Fan Page: cmberkeleymediagroup
Website: www.cmberkeleymediagroup.com
Email: info@cmberkeleymediagroup.com

Check out other great titles from our authors

For Adults

Eating4Eternity: Unlock Your Holistic Health Lifestyle.
Amazon Link >> http://amzn.to/1cO0kFd

Sweet Raw Desserts: Life Is Sweet Raw™
Amazon Link >> http://amzn.to/19msz2E

Can I Offer You A Cigarette: The Only Sure Way To Break The Smoking Habit
Amazon Link >> http://amzn.to/1enAfiJ

Colon By Design: Overcoming The Stigma Of Colon Sickness And Unlocking True Colon Health™
Amazon Link >> http://amzn.to/JGH05a

Fresh Food4Life™: The Case For Taking Back Control of Your Food And Empowering Your Family And Community.
Amazon Link >> http://amzn.to/J9yrQF

For Teens and Young Adults

The Youth Leadership Empowerment System™
Try out the FREE mini-course for youth.
Amazon Link >> http://amzn.to/1hRtMPy

For Children

The adventures of Moshe Monkey and Elias Froggy book series.

The Adventures of Moshe Monkey and Elias Froggy: A Healthy Business (Volume 1)
Amazon Link >> http://amzn.to/18V4NKO

Moshe and Elias Build A Garden (The Adventures of Moshe Monkey and Elias Froggy) (Volume 2)
Amazon Link >> http://amzn.to/1cj7elb

Moshe and Elias Tropical Vacation (The Adventures of Moshe Monkey and Elias Froggy) (Volume 3)
Amazon Link >> http://amzn.to/1hb1py7

For more great info from the author, fun activities for your children, and more, visit: http://mosheandelias.com

* * * * *

Want to become a published author in 90 days? CM Berkeley Media Group has an online training program to help anyone aspiring to achieve this dream. Find out more about it and realize your dream at
http://cmberkeleymediagroup.com/writeyourbookin90days/

Already have your manuscript written and want to work with us to turn your book into a kindle reality? We have services to help you polish your work, design the cover, and get your book formatted for kindle and print too. To get started visit our website at http://www.cmberkeleymediagroup.com

Great Resources

EternityWatch Magazine (www.eternitywatchmagazine.com)

EternityWatch Magazine is the premier magazine for those seeking a truly holistic approach to health and wellness. The magazine is founded on the belief that good health is everyone's birthright and that by proper education, people can make the right choices to maintain their good health. The magazine is focused on plant-based nutrition, thus it caters to the rapidly growing vegan, and raw/living foods movement. You can get it free online just by signing up for it.

Eating4Eternity.org (www.eating4eternity.org)

Eating4Eternity is founded by Jenny Berkeley and is focused on her personal coaching approach. On the site, you will find news articles on health and wellness, Jenny's blog posts with her personal insights into what is happening in the medical field, paid courses and webinars, and some free information.

FreshFood4Life.com (www.freshfood4life.com)

Fresh food for life is part of living a healthy life. This website has information about a revolutionary garden solution for the home owner with no space. You can view videos, articles and order your own garden system. You can grow 24 crops in you very own kitchen. I have one of these and so can you.

Hippocrates Health Institute (www.hippocratesinst.org)

Hippocrates Health Institute is the premier institute for alternative health and wellness. With over 50 years of experience in educating people to take control of their health destiny, the institute has a solid foundation. Their website talks about their programs, plus you can find copies of their magazine.

**CM Berkeley Media Group
(www.cmberkeleymediagroup.com)**
This is the website for anyone interested in becoming an
author. It contains some great insights into the writing
industry, resources for new authors, and an online course to
teach you how to write your book in 90 days. I use the
techniques in the course to help enhance my system for
writing my books. The course is worth 10 times what they
charge for it.

* * * * *

For Your Personal Notes

www.ingramcontent.com/pod-product-compliance
Lightning Source LLC
Chambersburg PA
CBHW071227290326
41931CB00037B/2232